E.A.T.

Evolve Advocate Transform

An Unconventional Decade In The Life Of A Cancer Patient

Kathy Mydlach Bero

Dedication

To EmmaGrace and Hannah who kept the light in my heart shining bright.

To Ron who used his juggling skills to manage every part of all our lives.

To Mom and Dad – there just are no words.

Foreword

Back in the days before children or sensible shoes, I was an avid Harley rider, taking my bike on tour, riding from show to show across the USA and beyond. While in Chicago, Illinois for U2's Zoo TV Tour, I had a couple of days off and only one thing on my mind – to make my way up to Milwaukee for a visit at the Harley-Davidson Motorcycle facility. I was lucky enough to meet with Bill Davidson and his father, Willie G., both of whom were very generous with their time. A highlight of that trip was having Willie G. show me how the company used his original drawings to create the finished product I had parked in my garage. Shortly after that visit, Bill invited me to join the Harley crew at the 1990 Daytona Bike Week. It was there that I met Ron and Kathy Bero who had been "assigned" by Bill, Ron's cousin, to keep me out of trouble. We became fast friends as we attempted to eat, sleep and drink all things Harley for the week. However, it was clear from the start that the beauty and efficiency of the new 'evolution engine' was not high on Kathy's list of topics to discuss. Instead, she opted to engage me in intense conversations ranging from the state of world politics to faith, and of course, the environment. It's fair to say that she approached each subject with polite determination, looking me straight in the eye, making sure every point was clearly understood. During one Daytona dinner, we became so engrossed in our own conversations that the rest of the party insisted we sit at opposite ends of the table, as if separating two bickering children. When I left Daytona Bike Week, I had realized a lifelong goal and made two new lifelong friends, and despite the geographical distance between us, we've managed to stay close.

In late 2005, Kathy called to break the impossible news that you never want to hear from a friend or family member. Kathy had been diagnosed with a rare and aggressive breast cancer, creating a benchmark in all our lives. I was terrified that Kathy's two young girls, EmmaGrace and Hannah, might lose her, and while I couldn't admit to it at the time, I felt entirely redundant, wanting to scream with frustration every time we hung up the phone. Then by coincidence, I came across the Angiogenesis Foundation (AF), a Massachusetts based non-profit organization promoting an anti-angiogenic treatment approach to chronic, inflammatory illnesses using specific foods, existing drugs and cutting edge medications. I called Kathy and regurgitated everything I could remember from what I had learned, including how a new drug called Avastin was showing promising results with certain types of cancers. Not one to shun potential weapons in her fight, Kathy agreed to let me put her in touch with Dr. Will Li, president

v

and medical director for the AF, who explained how adding anti-angiogenic compounds to her treatment regime could potentially help her beat cancer.

Having little time for self-pity, Kathy never revealed the full extent of the toll cancer treatment took on her, but ultimately due to her own self-advocacy, she received the best treatment available and is willing to tell her story for the benefit of all. As long as I've known Kathy, she has taken the focus off her own challenges by applying her skills to help others. Her battle with cancer was no different! During her recovery, Kathy founded NuGenesis, the first of its kind non-profit organization, which demonstrated another successful example of her tenacity to work for the greater good. She designed NuGenesis to teach patients and their families how to use food as medicine at every meal, and while her idea was simple, it took an enormous amount of time and energy. I know it was a labor of love, but it came at great personal cost for her.

Kathy Bero's story is a powerful one about stepping out in faith, embracing fears, and in a few clever Judo moves, turning the fear process on its head and into a force for good. Now, she's sharing her strategy with all of us.

--Larry Mullen, Jr., Founder U2

Revelation

April 2005

At 43, my husband, Ron, was tall and sinewy, carrying very little body fat on his ultra-marathon runs. In his first 100-mile race, Ron finished with a time of 19 hours and 35 minutes, placing him 95th of the nation's fastest ultra-runners. Meanwhile at 41, I struggled to recover from two pregnancies. Once fit, I was finding it hard to walk a couple of miles without collapsing from profound fatigue. I obsessed over my accelerated aging and was flummoxed by Ron's ability to defy his own. I wished he would scale back to accommodate my new physical state of motherhood, but he was literally leaving me in the dust, and its grit was thick in my mouth every day.

In our life before children we defined ourselves as the "wilderness adventure couple." Our entire relationship was built around rock climbing, mountain biking, skiing, canoeing, hiking, spelunking, ice climbing and sea kayaking. Encounters with bears, whales and the occasional wolf were par for the course. When at home, our entertainment included scanning the catalogues for the latest, greatest camping, climbing or paddling gear we just couldn't live without. It was gear we even found a use for in our home. For example, we used our climbing equipment to renovate a 150-year-old home and stabilize a bouncy 2nd floor bedroom above the sagging living room ceiling. Ron procured a 400-pound support beam and rigged our climbing ropes up with carabineers to install it onto a set of vertical posts he had notched out and fastened on either end of the 25-foot room. We hoisted that massive beam horizontally against the ceiling, bracing ourselves to maintain control as it swung on its tenuous line, coming inches from knocking a hole through the outside of the house and aiming to kill us on its way. I joined Ron in swearing a blue streak, grunting with sweat dripping in our eyes, down our arms and into our hands, causing the rope to slide through our slippery grip. I squeezed my grip tighter, which had been strengthened from untold hours of rock climbing, and managed to hold on as Ron delicately maneuvered the old timber, completing its placement. Heaving breaths, we stepped back to admire our work.

"It's fine," Ron said with a grin, admiring the strength of his partner and wife.

It always was. It seemed no matter what challenge we were confronted with, we always ended up just fine.

On one of my favorite expeditions, we kayaked the Kenai Fjords of Alaska. In August of 1996, we arrived in Seward as newly certified kayakers, having passed a simple test in the tepid waters of Waubesa Lake located in Madison, Wisconsin. Our footsteps clomped across the unevenly worn and weather-battered wooden dock at Port Seward as we approached the outfitter's raggedy shack to register. Inside the tiny crooked room, life jackets and paddles lined the walls. We showed our kayak certification, signed a waiver clearing them of any and all responsibility should we get injured or die, and paid for our rented kayaks and shuttle service to the drop off point. In the calm lake waters of Wisconsin, tipping over and pulling the spray skirt off while submerged underwater or rolling the boat back upright without exiting brought on fits of joy and laughter. It never even occurred to us how those same tasks would become dreadfully dangerous in the hypothermic-inducing waters we were about to navigate. The man running the outfitter was well-seasoned in the fishing industry. He wore torn and tattered, dirty, navy blue trousers and a grease-stained zip-up Carhartt jacket. He cared little about who we were or what we were doing and expressed no responsibility for informing us of the impending dangers we were about to encounter in those frigid North Pacific seas. That's how it was in Alaska – live and let live.

The following morning without so much as a hello, the deck hands strapped our kayaks to the racks on the shuttle, and as if exuberant puppies we joyfully followed with our bright yellow waterproof bags wobbling at our sides. Moments later, the choreographed crew unleashed the boat from the dock, pushed it off, jumped on and took their positions for the three-and-a-half-hour ride to Aialik Bay. There, we would spend the entire week paddling in the shadow of four receding glaciers while we explored the foreboding landscape of the fjords.

As soon as the boat left the bay at Seward, a pod of killer whales porpoised, flanking the boat. I leaned over the bow smiling ear to ear and snapped picture after picture, bending my knees to absorb every bump while shielding my camera from the rhythmic spray of the ocean. My body worked hard to stay balanced as the shuttle raced through the choppy sea colliding with each wave like a wrecking ball against a cement wall.

The captain calmly called to me, "If you fall in, you're not coming back."

My smile dropped, and my heart sank. Without pause I quickly moved in against the saltwater corroded cabin of the boat. I tucked my camera away and watched the whales through my God-given lenses. When we arrived at the ice-lined fjords, the captain unloaded our boats on a non-descript shore before backing up and out and giving us a farewell salute. There was no one there to greet us and no information kiosk or wooden map to point us in the right direction. Once the shuttle boat disappeared, we were on our own with no way back until he returned seven days later. It was absolutely exhilarating. We organized our gear into the hull of our small, narrow kayaks and paddled smoothly through the silty grey, ice-filled waters of the bay. Instantly, I felt tiny. The landscape rose sharply around us, and I found myself mesmerized as I stared down through the layers of gelatinous jellyfish drifting under and around our boats, popping and floating through the abyss of their liquid universe. We propelled ourselves past small icebergs as we struggled to approach Aialik Glacier, whose arctic winds kicked up powerful waves repelling our tiny boats.

My biceps burned as I skillfully dug deep into the paddler's strokes, swiftly steering clear of the enormous blocks of buoyant blue ice that had calved from the glacier's edge. When they crashed into the water, huge surface waves teetered my boat closer to flipping than I cared to experience, and while the orcas from the open sea were not visible in the fjord, with each and every wave, the thought of turning face down into an infestation of jellyfish sent a jolt of adrenaline through my body. With every stroke I worked to brace my boat against the surface of the water and slowly picked my way across the bay, singing out to calm my nerves. "Slow and steady wins the race."

Adventures like those renewed my spirit but were put on hold with the pregnancy of my first daughter, EmmaGrace. I was not good at being pregnant. I could climb a mountain with an 80-pound pack on my back while scanning the landscape for bears but struggled with another life growing inside my womb. For me, birth was in a whole different league of endurance activities. By the time my second daughter was born, I moved through each day bedraggled, barely remembering my adventures let alone considering taking part in one.

Exhaustion dogged me each day. Something wasn't right. Something was happening in my body, but I didn't have a name for it. I was generally a "go with the flow" kind of person but became frustrated and wanted out of that flow. I felt like a tethered dog spying a bunny across the yard. Every time I tried to race forward and reclaim some part of my previous existence, an invisible chain jerked me back so hard my bones hit against my organ-filled cavity with a thud. I so badly wanted to get back out into life, but my lack of energy left me shackled in a heap on the living room couch.

Then came the day Ron noticed my hair in the shower drain.

Spring 2005
My second daughter, Hannah, was 18 months old when I decided to ignore my weakening state and forge ahead by grabbing a dream 23 years in the making. I wanted to herd sheep with my border collies. The time had come. We had our farm. We had a fenced five-acre pasture where a small flock of sheep would live with our two rescued cows and two horses. The sheep would be delivered at the end of the summer after my dog and I had completed our first round of training.

I joined the Wisconsin Working Stock Dog Association (WWSDA) and enrolled in three sheep herding clinics run by some of the top herders in the world. My pup, Albert, was a star. At just 10 months old, his furry, black-and-white spotted frame was very muscular. He had a keen eye and a strong work ethic. He was a playful family dog who loved to chase balls and wrestle with his favorite chew toy – a ring of primary-colored plastic keys. But when Albert saw the chickens at the edge of our yard, a switch was thrown. His head lowered as his front legs dropped to a crouch position, and his eyes darted from the chickens to me as if to beg, "Can I move them? Can I? Can I? Can I?"

In my mind, there was nothing more impressive than sending a dog out into a lush green valley towards a small flock of white sheep speckling the turf a half of a mile away. In herding competitions, the good shepherd directed her dog with a few short whistles to move the flock towards a small pen waiting at the other end of the field. Just like at a golf tournament, the audience at those trials spoke in hushed tones as the tension built with every deliberate step the determined dog took. Its eyes locked on each sheep, stalking the edges of the flock and watching for one to break. The sheep crowded nervously together gingerly prancing as they moved closer to the gate. There was no way for them to escape the intense eye of the border collie. So, resigned to their fate, they shoved past each other into the pen. The shepherd, who always stood calmly at the ready, waited with the gate in hand for that exact moment when all of the sheep were in and then slammed the gate shut. Time! The crowd cheered, and the shepherd praised her dog who continued to pace in a crouched position around the pen with its primal predatory instincts fully engaged and ready to complete the kill. While maneuvering a herd of sheep, the border collie's riveting display of extreme self-control demonstrated an impressive exhibition of a mock hunt.

Albert was ready. Me? Well, let's just say Albert carried me. He did everything he could to make me look good. I imagined it was frustrating for

4

him, but he wanted to herd in the worst way and remained the consummate professional. He would subtly swiped a look at me and then in mid-crouch focused his eyes in the direction he wanted to take the sheep. Finally, putting two and two together, I realized that when he took my lead, the sheep scattered. So, I got better at taking his. Without any help from me, Albert moved the flock in fluid unison as I waved my stick around periodically saying, "There" or "Lie down" just to make it look as if I wasn't a deadbeat shepherd. Who was I kidding?

I had planned to enter our first novice trial later that spring at a beautiful farm in the Baraboo Hills of Wisconsin. The site was reminiscent of inland Scotland where the shepherds sent their dogs out for miles to collect the sheep and safely return them to their shepherd's barn yard. In Baraboo, the fields were much smaller, but it was still the quintessential border collie haven. The hues of green on the landscape provided a stunning backdrop for the black and white dogs moving waves of white, wooly sheep over the hills and valleys speckled with apple trees. During the trials, some truly exceptional shepherds casually steered their dogs with short whistles to signal them to make direction changes, and then leaned on their crooks to chat with the course minders or admiring audience lining the hillside opposite the penning gate. In preparation for the competition, Albert and I attended a three-day clinic. The instructor, Julie Simpson, came all the way from Scotland. The only woman to ever win the Supreme International Championship had somehow found her way to Spooner, Wisconsin, to coach our little herding club in the art of natural dog handling. She was, as they say, the supreme alpha dog. Everyone wanted to please her, including me.

It was an incredible opportunity, but the nagging fatigue plagued me all weekend as I struggled to engage. The shadow of something sinister lurking in my body followed me everywhere I went. After every shower, I picked out the tangled clumps of my long, curly blonde hair clogging the hotel drain. I urgently guzzled cranberry juice whenever I could get it even though its tart dryness was never a favorite in my mouth. Without realizing it, I was witnessing the proverbial tip of the iceberg as it surfaced.

A few weeks later, I found a small red spot on my thigh and dismissed it as a bug bite, but its persistence drove me to visit a dermatologist who diagnosed me with Lyme disease and immediately started me on a five-day course of antibiotics. Each day, I studied the spot looking for any signs of change, but there were none.

June 2005

Too busy, too stubborn and in a state of unconscious denial, I ignored the aching spot on my leg and went to another herding clinic with my friend Ann. When I bent over to pick up a box out of the car trunk, she immediately noted the red streak moving up my thigh and disappearing under my shorts. Alarmed, she pleaded with me to leave the clinic and go straight to the hospital, which forced me to say that I would even though I knew I wouldn't. Throughout the day, the itchy, hot, prickly pain tracked up my leg firing a static charge just under the skin. I tried to brush it away, but relief was elusive. At the end of the day, instead of honoring my word, I went straight home to celebrate my first-born's graduation from first grade.

EmmaGrace had a passion for camping and wanted to hold her graduation party in our black walnut grove where we could roast hot dogs and marshmallows over the fire, tell stories and sing songs. The celebratory night faded as our energy waned. We sat in the swing chairs Ron had suspended under the canopy of towering trees and listened to the droning croaks of frogs in the adjacent marsh. Our silence gave way to the crickets who took over the darkened stage as our domed red tent beckoned us to bed. So, with droopy eyes, we tucked ourselves in, and everyone drifted off to sleep…except me.

In a matter of minutes, I began tossing and turning with the itching pain burning out of control and moving into my torso. Exhausted and frenzied, I quietly crawled over the bodies of my sleeping family and bolted from the tent to hide in the comfort of my own bed where I slept fitfully throughout the night. By morning, I lay in agony on our antique, pea green couch, shifting uncomfortably around the lumps of matted cotton stuffing when Ron and the girls wandered in from outside. I looked up from the couch and weakly met Ron's dark blue eyes, which instantly filled with alarm. Dripping wet, it was obvious I had spiked a very high fever. He forcefully pronounced that it was time to go to the hospital, and even if I had had the energy, how could I have argued?

I was dismayed that I hadn't listened to Ann. Ron packed up food and toys for the girls and schlepped their stuff and their mother to the ER. I lamented my stupidity, having waited until Sunday to see a doctor, which most likely meant we'd have a long wait in the triage area. When we arrived, I dragged myself through the sliding doors of the admittance area and found a happy surprise. There was only one other person waiting. He was dressed in ripped up jeans and a torn, mud-smeared, red tartan flannel shirt. His arms and face were bloody, and he held an ice pack to his head. The man, in his 50s, had been putting a new roof on his house when he slipped on a loose shingle and slid

6

off, falling hard to the planting below. I felt bad for him as he sat slouched in his wheel chair looking pretty demoralized. To me, it seemed obvious that he would be called before me, but when the ER nurse appeared at the swinging doors, she called my name instead.

The highly skilled ER team at our little Oconomowoc Memorial Hospital was consistently ranked at the top of emergency rooms in the country. Their quick diagnosis of a lymphatic staph infection set in motion a flurry of activity during which they inserted a catheter into my arm and pumped high doses of intravenous antibiotics through my veins. As I passively lay there watching them prep my arm, the kids squirmed, and Ron turned away.

I told them, "It's no biggy. Needles don't worry me. This is nothing – piece of cake." Then, I sang a section from little Hannah's favorite Disney Halloween song, "They Can't Scare Me!"

I smiled a sincere and convincing smile at my girls unaware that it would be only a few short months before I would become extremely needle-phobic and not able to honestly muster that song ever again.

While the infection resolved fairly quickly, I continued to battle fatigue and hair loss. One problem after another provided clues to my failing health, but doctors of all disciplines struggled to pinpoint the problem.

In an effort to lift my spirits, Ron pronounced, "You're fine. Let's start up date night again."

He was good at that – pronouncing. It was how he dealt with stress. It was nice in theory, but I had trouble mustering up the energy to even sit upright let alone go out on a date. My motivation was in the crapper, and all I wanted to do was sleep, but like every other mother with small children, I brushed it off.

August 2005
Each day, I looked out the kitchen window to spy my two horses who always seemed to be staring back from the fence. They were used to regular attention from me, and my guilt over neglecting them weighed heavy. They spent their days grazing in the pasture, whether they were bored or thrilled was hard to say. Horses truly are naturally lazy, but ours seemed to like interacting with us; otherwise, I don't think they would have run to the fence whenever we approached. I consoled myself by focusing on the five-acre pasture, two cows and flock of chickens keeping them company and allowed myself to relax.

7

Simon was my favorite. He was a Government Morgan bred to work. I thought of him as the border collie of the horse world. We met at the boarding facility where I was riding and learning equine husbandry before EmmaGrace and Hannah were even a glimmer of a thought. When I first saw Simon, who was brought there to be sold, he was just a terrified three-year-old pacing in his temporary stall. Although he was so young, Simon had already endured physical abuse delivered at the hand of his breeder, and with larger-than-life eyes, he drew me in. Even though I knew very little about taking care of horses, I purchased him in the spirit of sparing him from any future hardships.

I used up all of my accumulated vacation time and spent five hours a day, six days a week getting to know my new horse. I brushed him, sang to him and played with him. We learned to trail ride together, and by the end of 1997, Simon seemed to know me better than I knew myself. When he began to nuzzle my belly with gentle pushes that made me giggle, the trainer at the barn cautioned me that he was being rude, but it didn't feel that way. Then one day, it occurred to me that I had missed my period. Simon wasn't shy with his love for babies no matter what the species, dividing his compassion equally between the youngest horses and puppies, moving gently around human children and even watching over a zebra in his pasture that had been rescued from the circus. So, one Saturday when Ron and I were on our way to shop for upgraded camping gear, I just had to find out if Simon knew something I didn't.

"I need to stop at Walgreens," I told Ron.

"Why?" he asked.

"I'll tell you after I get what I need," I responded evasively.

Ron pulled into the parking lot, and I launched out of the car and scurried in through the doors laughing out loud at myself. I found the aisle with the pregnancy tests, bought one and ducked into the bagel shop next store. In their bathroom, I read the instructions carefully then followed them closely. As I counted the seconds, two lines materialized in the oval window at the end of the plastic stick. I read the directions again, which clearly stated that one line was negative, two lines were positive. The lines were fairly faint, and I wondered if my eyes were playing tricks on me. Did I really see two lines, or was the color bleeding through from the moisture? Uncertainty morphed into certainty. A huge smile filled my face as joy welled up from my heart. I was pregnant and in a split second I was overflowing with love for that little baby. I laughed all the way back to the car.

"It's positive!" I said through hearty laughter.

I waved the pregnancy test in the air and said it again, "It's positive! I'm pregnant!"

I watched as Ron's dumbfounded expression changed to understanding followed by happiness and then elation.

"We're having a baby?" he asked rhetorically.

Thursday, October 27, 2005

Simon did it again in 2003 with my second pregnancy. He was two for two, but when he started pushing at my right breast less than two years later, I didn't make the connection. I thought he was getting pushy because I felt so weak. I knew I wasn't pregnant again because Ron's tubes were tied. So, the only logical conclusion was that I must've entered menopause. I had always developed faster than my peers, and it would seem that I was entering mid-life faster as well. I was an old lady, and Simon mostly only liked babies.

So, the evening of October 27, 2005 was a watershed moment when Simon's true motive was revealed. While drying off after a shower, I noticed a small, dime-sized red spot on my chest. As if I was standing in a powerful ocean surf, a wave of fear knocked me back. My first thought was to run outside and hug Simon. He wasn't being pushy at all he was telling me I was sick. He had done what the doctors couldn't. It was another "Lassie" moment similar to the time when I woke up one Sunday morning in 1998 to a voicemail informing me that Simon had been taken to a large horse show by the trainer who boarded him. EmmaGrace was just six months old, and my visits to Simon were unpredictable, so the trainer assumed I wouldn't be there and had "taken" him to a show without my permission. That was the word she used on the message. She just took – kidnapped – my horse. She thought she could earn a little commission by finding a buyer at the show and then convince me to sell Simon, "what with the baby and all."

On that Sunday morning, my head was so hot I could feel the steam pouring out of my eyes and ears as I ran out of the door yelling to Ron, "You're in charge!"

Then I raced to rescue Simon. The show was at the Jefferson County Fairgrounds in a huge outbuilding filled with portable stalls holding hundreds of horses. I stood at the open end of the building scanning the crowds of people impeccably clad in jodhpurs, English-styled shirts and leather riding boots. I didn't recognize anyone and clearly did not fit, looking disheveled in my sweats and helplessly enraged. I didn't know what else to do but call out.

"SIMON!" I hollered as loudly as I could.

It only took a second for his ear-piercing whinny to carry through the cavernous building buzzing with activity. He whinnied again, and I followed his call, picking my way through the narrow aisles careful not to trip on the farrier tools, tack trunks, coolers and grain buckets scattered around each stall. At the far end, I found Simon sweaty and scared, pacing on a small piece of concrete surrounded by moveable stall walls. The trainer, who stole my boy, was nowhere in sight. As I led him through the crowds and out of the building, walking seemed to calm his nerves. I loaded him onto the trailer and drove him to a friend's farm just down the road from mine., and that's where he stayed until our barn was ready for my "Lassie" to come home.

Dragging myself back from happy memories, I looked at myself in the mirror and gingerly touched the red spot on top of a 25-year-old scar where a benign cyst had been removed. I felt a small something, but not really anything. The area was warm, but then again, I had just gotten out of the shower. A flash of electricity ran through my body. Even though I couldn't feel anything defined, it was there. The soft, elusive mass seemed to dissipate under my touch. I was overwhelmed by a tsunami of fear before wave after wave of clarity rolled over my mind, leaving me with no doubt as to what it was. What else could it be? I had been poked, prodded and examined for everything else. My head was on fire, and my body flushed with panic and felt anchored by lead as my heartbeat clobbered at my temples. I was overwhelmed with the adrenaline of dread, and a chorus of every cell in my body screamed the unthinkable, "YOU HAVE CANCER!"

Standing alone in the bathroom with everyone else asleep, I took a deep breath in and stared at myself in the mirror. The black and white subway tiles on the walls faded from view, and all I could see was that red spot reflected back at me through the steam. My body knew what was growing inside and had been sending me messages all along, but I had been too busy to hear the alarm bells signaling cancer. Thank God Simon hadn't been.

As my brain re-engaged, the adrenaline dissipated. I thought about waking Ron and telling him I had cancer, but I knew he would just dismiss me with, "You're fine. There's no way you could have cancer. What would the odds of that be?" I didn't know what the odds were then, but I do now. One in seven women would be diagnosed with breast cancer that year, and those weren't very good odds for me. Instead, I phoned Suzannah, Ron's sister and a physician's assistant (PA) at Memorial Sloan-Kettering. After I described what I had found, the dismay in her silent pause was palpable.

"Oh, Kath," she blurted out.

Then, as if a switch had been thrown, she became compassionately professional and described the possibilities. It was clear from Suzannah's voice that it was not good, but I had no idea just how "not good" it really was. She asked me to get paper and pen to write down the very specific instructions she was about to give me. At the top of the list for the next morning was to go directly to my OBGYN and not leave until I had undergone each test she named. Suzannah, my own personal PA, presented me with the dialogue that would unfold and gave me the words I had to use to get where I needed to go.

"Those symptoms are typical of an infection," she said in a deep deadpan tone. "That's most likely what it is, but don't leave until you've had a physical exam, a mammogram and an ultrasound. Have them fax all the results to me right away. If anything shows up, I'll have you schedule the appropriate biopsy."

Suzannah knew they would want to give me antibiotics and send me home, assuming I had mastitis, an infection in my mammary ducts. She was certain this was not the case and sternly instructed me to stay until I had completed all the tests. Not generally a pessimist, I assumed she thought I "only" had the regular curable breast cancer. I had no idea there were 30 different types, and without naming it out loud, Suzannah had diagnosed me with the rare and difficult to diagnose, inflammatory breast cancer. I hung up the phone and began rifling through my memory bank trying to find what I had recently read or heard about breast cancer and its rates of survival. I thought it was 98% of all breast cancers were curable. After all my grandmother had been diagnosed with breast cancer when she was in her early 70's. She had a successful mastectomy with no other treatment and died 20 years later happy and fulfilled. I took her memory to bed with me and lay in the darkness persuading myself I would be fine too.

The minutes ticked by but sleep was elusive. Controlling my destiny was my preferred state of being, but a diagnosis of cancer left me completely out of control. There would be no plucking the tumor from my chest, tossing it in the trash and going along my merry way. In the darkness, my thoughts turned to Suzannah and how dependent I had just become on my "little sister."

11

Friday, October 28, 2005

When morning finally broke, I woke Ron and filled his groggy head with the previous night's events. In a mild state of shock, he drove the girls to school as he normally did. I called my OBGYN, Dr. Tousignant, who first took me in as a patient when I was surprised, elated and then scared witless by my first pregnancy. Two weeks early, EmmaGrace arrived on Dr. Tousignant's day off, but staying true to her promise to deliver my baby, she came racing in on her Harley-Davidson. She swooped into my birthing room dressed in her riding clothes and caught my crowing baby just in the nick of time.

On the phone with Dr. Tousignant's office and armed with Suzannah's list of tests, I froze when they told me she was not in. I was blasted with a chill that ran down my spine, spreading throughout my entire body before sending the same deep freeze through the telephone wires. The assistant quickly added that the PA would be happy to see me as soon as I could get there. I hung up, looked out the kitchen window and saw that Ron had just pulled into the driveway. I grabbed my instructions from Suzannah and ran out to the car.

On the way to the doctor's, I rehearsed what I needed to say. I was so grateful for Suzannah's coaching, which allowed me to push back at the paralyzing fear welling up from the depths of my soul. That first lesson in self-advocacy was the biggest gift she could've given me. Without her words, I would've ended up like so many women who were put on hold and told to "come back in six months unless something changes." For the cancer growing in my body, six months longer would've put me six feet under.

Ron parked the car in the hospital garage, and we made our way to the door. Our footsteps echoed as we descended the concrete stairwell to the street level where we crossed the driveway in front of the hospital, moved through the electric doors and stepped onto the elevator. Not wanting to meet anyone's eyes, I kept my head down, never glancing up. On the third floor, the elevator doors opened. We stepped out into a nondescript hall and turned right to Dr. Tousignant's door just a few feet from the elevator. In the waiting room, I slipped into a corner chair, and Ron checked me in.

"How could this happen to me?" I thought to myself.

Swirling around and around in my head, that question jumped like a ping-pong ball off my angry paddle to my scared paddle, hit my sad paddle and ricocheted back to my even angrier paddle. I had been healthy for 41 years. I ate well, exercised regularly and lived a very clean life. I never smoked

12

and even covered my mouth at the gas station to filter the benzene fumes while I filled the tank.

I repeated that monologue over and over at high speed in my head as my legs bounced. I glanced at the other patients, hoping to find something familiar to cling to. Most looked tired but joyful with babies in their bellies or sleeping next to them secured in car seats on the floor. When one woman caught my eye I froze, prickling with embarrassment. I was sure I recognized pity emanating from her compassionate gaze, and I was paranoid that she knew I would soon be diagnosed. My dad had always encouraged us to be strong and resilient, but all I felt at that moment was vulnerable and weak. I was miserably self-conscious having been violated by the evil growing in my body. I quickly averted my eyes from her and studied the matted threads of the blue carpet at my feet as if the cure was held captive in the nap. I was stressed and sleep deprived, which made the entire scene seem almost surreal. I forced myself to switch my subject of interest to other items in the room and found familiar photos of flowers arranged in serene settings evenly spaced on the walls. When I realized that my friend Janet had taken each one, I was afforded a millisecond of happiness. Losing myself in that little moment of engineered serenity, I didn't hear the nurse call my name from the threshold of the door to the exam rooms. Ron took my hand and snapped me back to my dismal reality.

"Kathy," she called again while standing in the open doorway, glancing down at my file to be sure she was calling the correct name.

I slowly got up from my chair and with my head down followed her through the hall until she motioned me into the exam room and closed the door behind me.

"Have a seat in one of these chairs and tell me what brought you here today," she directed.
I sat obediently in the familiar chairs and began to read from my instructed notes.

"I found a spot on my right breast last night, and my sister-in-law, who is in breast cancer and melanoma at Memorial Sloan-Kettering, sent me to have a series of tests today," I said and then paused, watching her face to measure her response.

Dr. Tousignant's PA jotted down some notes, stood and asked, "Can you please put this gown on with the opening to the front? I'll wait right outside."

13

My shoulders dropped. I took the gown from her and smiled weakly as she stepped out of the room. As soon as she shut the door, I sighed. I knew what to do but resisted once again trying to understand what was happening. With a heavy sigh, I changed into the crinkly white paper gown, swatting it down along my body as I sat on the exam table just as she knocked at the door to come back in.

"Let's take a look at the spot you're concerned about," she said patting the table and motioning me to lie back.

She studied the spot, did a breast exam and then reached out her hand to pull me up.

"It looks like mastitis, which is an infection in your mammary duct. Are you still nursing?" she asked.

"No. My youngest is 18 months old," I responded.

She pulled out her prescription pad and wrote up an order for antibiotics just as protocol had dictated, and I pocketed the prescription.

"Now, I need to have a mammogram," I told her feeling a little stronger.

She opened my chart, scanned it for a few seconds and said, "You just had one six months ago. There was nothing suspicious found at that time, so it's not likely to have changed."

"I know, but my sister-in-law said I need another one, so please organize that for me," I said more sternly leaving her no way to decline.

With no discernable reaction, she obliged and led me through a muddy pink-colored, institutional corridor that led to the women's center where I was asked to change again into a thick, cozy white terrycloth robe meant to frame the experience in a spa-like setting. Of course, they missed the mark. Instead of peaceful, I felt vulnerably exposed as I proceeded sheepishly into the low light waiting room.

I waited only a few minutes for the ultrasound technician dressed in green hospital scrubs to fetch me, and with an unnaturally cheery demeanor, she escorted me to the mammography room down the hall. The scan itself lasted only a few minutes, but it was physically and mentally grueling. My breast was lifted onto the clear plastic plate, and then another plate was brought

14

down on top, squeezing me to a thickness of an inch or two. It was terrifying, and all I could think about was "pop" goes the tumor as I held my breath hoping to stand still enough to ensure the process wouldn't have to be repeated.

With only a moment's delay, the radiologist popped in the room, and I stood to receive her verdict.

She announced with a smile that, "Like the ones before, the new results are also negative."

I felt my knees buckle and almost collapsed from relief. For a brief second, I considered going home, but Suzannah's strict marching orders replayed loudly in my head. Her instructions became a mantra of sorts to help me avoid a misdiagnosis.

I began again, "My sister, Suzannah, is a physician's assistant in breast cancer and melanoma at Memorial Sloan-Kettering, and she said I am to have an ultrasound next."

In truth, Suzannah had moved to North Carolina just a couple months before but still maintained all of her contacts and relationships at the top cancer hospital in the country, and in my mind, she was still there. When I met Suzannah, she was just five years old and I was a senior in high school, dating her brother Ron. She was full of life, perpetually running with her tight, wild curls bouncing in the air and her blue eyes smiling as wide as her mouth. She was always laughing and looking for hugs, leaving me captivated by her joy and energy. Suzannah was a compassionate, positive and self-confident girl; and as she grew into a woman, her many skills and talents were clearly evident. Her tenacity to conquer challenges was undeniably impressive. In Indiana's Little 500 bicycle race, she suffered an excruciating fall on the cinder track, and with blood streaming down her bruised limbs, Suzannah still managed to help carry her college team on to victory. Some eight years later, she would become my champion as well and hopefully lead me on to triumph over cancer.

Each medical professional I encountered throughout that first day was respectfully accommodating and willing to follow Suzannah's orders. So, it was off to the ultrasound room three doors down. While prepping my skin with a warm gel and then moving the ergonomically designed wand over my breast tissue, the ultrasound technician lightly chatted with me in the darkened room, joking and catching up on her wedding ring saga. After the positive mammogram results, I was allayed and laughed a little too hard at her story. Laura was the person who had done my previous mammogram, during which she shared the tale of how her fiancé had been ripped off by the jeweler who sold him a flawed engagement ring. Since then, they had gotten married and found the whole debacle laughable. We giggled some more about it and then hit a snag. Her smiling face went flat. She swiped the ultrasound wand over the red spot another time, and I knew something was wrong. My eyes widened, and my body bristled with fear. Laura moved the wand to my side and pushed uncomfortably hard to get deeper into the tissue while punching keys on her computer to mark the offending area on the screen. When she was done, she handed me a washcloth to wipe the blue gel from my skin and with a faltering smile, said she would be back after the radiologist had taken a look at my pictures.

I cleaned up, and instead of staying on the table, I moved to the chair trying to look like a normal person. I didn't ask for this new position in life and completely rejected the notion that I was a cancer patient, even though I clearly was. I felt entirely undignified in that standard-issue gown and wanted to get dressed to call my hospital's bluff and hold on to "normal" a little bit longer. I leafed through outdated *People* magazines, forcing interest as if "They" were watching to see how I was handling the strain and thinking about how "They" would break the news. By the time I moved on to reading about politics in *TIME*, the radiologist finally gave the obligatory knock at the door, opening it before I could even answer. She wore a muted smile and got right down to it.

"So, there is an area between 1.2 – 1.5 centimeters in size that gives me cause for concern. I'd like to do a biopsy as soon as possible., and since this is Friday, I'd like to schedule you right away on Monday morning. I'll have my scheduler arrange that for you," she said not meaning it as a suggestion.

The adrenaline rushed to my head, flushing my face and then sweat broke out on my forehead. I didn't want to panic. I had plans on Monday and didn't want to change them. The day after, I had a field trip to the zoo scheduled with my daughter. No, that wasn't going to work, I thought. I had no time for more tests, let alone cancer.

"I won't be able to come back until next Friday," I responded thinking I might be ready by then.

"Are you sure you don't want to do this sooner?" she asked with the very clear suggestion that I did.

"Yes," I answered quickly and stood up to end the conversation.

Truthfully, I wasn't sure. All I was sure about was that I needed to breathe the fresh air outside. I needed to privately feel sorry for myself. I needed to cry in the security of my own vehicle, and I needed to live.

Later that afternoon, I apprehensively called Suzannah to let her know I hadn't scheduled the biopsy right away, but mercifully, she didn't question me. Her professionally unambiguous support took me by surprise and felt very unfamiliar. Having worked with many women in my position, she graciously offered to answer all of my questions and left it at that. I think I thanked her and said I needed to "just let everything go for a few days." Let it go? I had no idea what I was talking about. I didn't know anyone that could let a cancer diagnosis "go," but I guess I just needed to try and stay in my current state of normal before the cruel grip of malignancy morphed me into something I didn't want to be – a cancer patient.

Saturday, October 29, 2005
It was Halloween weekend, our favorite holiday, and we meandered after EmmaGrace through the neighborhoods as she ran unbridled from house to house dressed as a Bratz Doll in full make-up, reveling in her huge "big girl" moment. Hannah was just two years old and was dressed as a glittery pink unicorn. She stumbled along trying to keep up with her sister, repeating over and over with a questioning smile, "Corn, Mommy?" It was absolutely joyful. She was in awe of the little bag of candy filling up as she presented it again and again to perfect strangers, but that wasn't even the best part. What blew her mind most was that she got to eat it at will. Ah, the simple joys of childhood! I made no room for cancer that night as I laughed with my family and chatted with friends. Cancer had no right to steal that joy from me, and I truly almost did let "it" go.

Sunday, October 30, 2005
The next night was a completely different story. Our friends Sheila and John had invited us to an adults-only costume party in Maple Bluff, a suburb of Madison, Wisconsin. We went as a hillbilly preacher and his wife, which didn't feel like much of a stretch since we lived on a farm and felt a little hillbilly at times with our 200 lb. Irish wolfhound lounging in the yard while chickens pecked at bugs a safe distance away. Unfortunately, the night was a bust for me. The shadow of the grim reaper followed me through every conversation. I feigned enjoyment, and no one seemed the wiser, but at one point, I became overwhelmed with fear. I slipped out through the front door and stood alone in the yard, hidden in the darkness, listening to my breath and crying. The questions poured through my mind

17

like corn from a silo.

"What is happening to me? How could I have cancer?" I directed my questions up to the heavens. "Is anyone there? Are you there, God? It's me, Kathy."

Memories from my past floated through like clouds ushering in a massive thunderstorm. I had spent my adult years working as a tireless advocate for the ecosystem, mostly focused on saving wild habitat and trying to get poisons out of our air and water. My ill-informed perception of cancer was that only smokers or people living in an environment compromised by industrial pollution were at risk, and that wasn't me. I lived on a 60-acre hobby farm. Our well was 250 feet deep, far out of the reach of any farm field run off. I ate fresh, healthy food and kept toxic cleaning supplies, if any, to a bare minimum in my house. I was living as poison free as I could.

I was hit with a memory from a few months earlier when my husband asked with a playful snicker, "What's with all of the hair in the shower drain, Hon? You're going to be bald before me!"

Neither one of us had any idea what he had predicted. I wasn't just going to lose some of my hair I was going to lose it all, including my eyebrows and eyelashes. Standing outside in the cold, dark Halloween air, I let out a gasp that turned to mist. I watched it linger for a moment and returned to the party.

November 4, 2005
Halloween celebrations came to an end, and I could no longer pretend I was fine. The day of my biopsy had arrived. I lay on the table with several monitor screens surrounding me. Some flashed light grey lines on a black screen and others glowed orange like the cursor on the computer screen at my first real job out of college. The technician unfolded a blue sheet from a stainless-steel tray, revealing the tools of the trade. A small pile of cotton swabs and a brownish yellow bottle of iodine sat beside each other ready to sanitize the surface of my skin. A purple marker would be used to draw dots to guide the radiologist's needle over the tumor. When I glanced at the cavernous biopsy needle sitting ominously on the tray, I felt repulsed and quickly turned my head away. I had only ever seen a needle that big for basting a turkey. My heart beat faster as the technician slid the blood pressure cuff over my arm. One of the dark screens to my left came to life and beeped as it registered my blood pressure - 148/87. Usually, it was very low, somewhere around 106/62, but my breathing had quickened, and sweat was once again beading on my forehead. Except to put the blood pressure

cuff on, not one human hand had even touched me yet. My fear was entirely based in the terrifying expectation of what was to happened. The technician glanced at my face, and with her lips compassionately pursed, she moved to the sink, wet a washcloth and placed it on my forehead to help cool and calm me down.

The radiologist entered the room with gloved hands held above her waist and away from her body and then asked, "Are you ready?"

I choked out, "Don't talk to me. Just go." Then, I gave a weak smile to make up for my rudeness, and she inserted the first needle.

It was tiny and sent lidocaine into my tissue deadening the nerves. After a minute or two, the technician laid the ultrasound wand on my breast, moving it at different angles to pick up the best view of the tumor. Once the white mass appeared on the screen, the radiologist picked up a larger needle, bent over my chest, glancing briefly at my face before plunging it deep into my tissue. I quickly turned my head away just in time to see the monitor opposite the doctor reveal the white needle penetrating the surface of my ethereal-looking tissue and piercing the surface of the tumor. It seemed counter intuitive to me. Wouldn't breaking the seal, so to speak, spread the cancer? I didn't dare speak. I just watched in horror as the needle was forced down into the mass, drawn out and reinserted at a different angle, leaving a trail reminiscent of jet exhaust crisscrossed through my breast tissue. In total the radiologist took five core samples from the tumor and put each one in a test tube with liquid to preserve it for the lab. Then, she asked me if I wanted to look at them. My relief was immediate.

I breathed. It was over. I took the washcloth off my head, sat up and looked at the vial. The scientist in me had emerged, and I felt detached from the samples of cylindrical breast tissue floating in the glass tube. I was fascinated by its lack of blood. They didn't look at all as I expected. They were whitish, worm-like entities somehow completely foreign to me, not black and nasty as I had imagined.

Monday, November 7, 2005
*"A vision without a task is but a dream, a task without a vision is drudgery, a vision and a task is the hope of the world." – **Anonymous***

Happily, time generously flew by, and on Monday, the results were in. My body was hosting an infiltrating ductal carcinoma. Dr. Tousignant called me with the results while I was driving in the car.

"Why don't you park the car, and then I can talk with you about the results of your biopsy?" she asked.

"Thanks, but I'm in a hurry to pick up Hannah. I know it's not good news, so go ahead and give it to me," I responded with a somewhat dismissive air.

I didn't want to slow down for cancer, but she insisted, so I parked.

"Your biopsy showed a fairly small tumor called an infiltrating ductal carcinoma," she said and then paused waiting for my response.

"I already know I have cancer," I said stupidly.

Dr. Tousignant continued, "I know you, Kathy. Treat it like a job, and you will get through it. I'll have my assistant call you later to organize an appointment with Dr. Doering. We affectionately call him the 'breast guy' because he's the only one any of our doctors would go to."

"Yeah. OK. Thanks for calling," I responded and then hung up the phone.

I shifted the car into reverse and backed out of the parking spot that had just served as a doctor's office. I paused for a minute and let out a breath, shifted into drive and slowly pulled up to the curb. Before the call, I had been rushing to pick Hannah up from day care, and after the call it felt like I was pushing my way through a glob of jelly. Even though it was a short conversation, I couldn't decide how I felt about it. Shaking off the gunk, I forced myself to focus on the task at hand and then pulled out into traffic to recover my sweet little baby girl.

Until recently, I had no idea how important Dr. Tousignant's simple words would be. They were the best advice she could've given me, and I've shared them many times with other women who have faced a similar road. For me her words were the point when flight turned to fight – the vision to beat cancer became my task.

The radiologist called to confirm the pathology report but added a caveat, which sucked the wind right out of my sails. She believed I had inflammatory breast cancer (IBC) but would need additional tests to confirm her suspicion. I felt indignant about what she said. My fear or perhaps ego caused me to feel that her comment was almost presumptuous. Suzannah hadn't even labelled the cancer yet, and my obstetrician had already given me the diagnosis. So, I chose to ignorantly focus on the lesser of two evils, the infiltrating ductal carcinoma and checked out the

20

Internet where I found a reference to a 89% cure rate. The treatment would be a lumpectomy, and that would be the end of it. It wouldn't be anything near the orthopedic operations I had been subjected to in the past. A lumpectomy seemed easy breezy by comparison.

"It's all good," I said reassuring myself.

I called Suzannah to report that the tumor was only a 1.5 centimeter infiltrating ductal carcinoma, but in the first second she spoke, I could almost smell the rubber burning on my braking tires.

"I agree with the radiologist. I'm certain you have IBC, and if that's the case, time is of the essence. You need to call Dr. Doering right when we hang up and go in for a skin punch biopsy and breast MRI immediately, which will confirm or deny our suspicions. IBC is quite rare, making up approximately 1% of all breast cancers, and most doctors don't know how to identify it until it's too late," Suzannah said in a very commanding and somewhat urgent tone.

She went on to explain how difficult IBC was to treat and that she would work with the doctors at Memorial Sloan-Kettering to put my plan together.

I called Ron, and all he could say was, "You'll be fine."

He's Mr. Positive and Mr. Denial rolled up into one. It's always a "fine" line with him.

That night, I took the girls to their swimming lessons at the YMCA and had plenty of time to think about my situation while I sat sweating on the bleachers in the pool area. Overwhelmed by the heat, I exploded into intense anger and couldn't shake it before the end of class. My change in mood must have been clearly evident to EmmaGrace. In the car on the way home she wisely asked me to put in a CD of my dad playing the piano. He was a self-taught, very accomplished musician, and for his birthday one year, my brother and I gave him a recording session at Smart Studios in Madison, Wisconsin. The last two songs we recorded were Christmas songs on which my dad accompanied our family chorus. I popped the CD in the narrow slot on my car radio and hit play. The songs melted through the speakers, dissipating my anger and causing tears to pour out from my eyes, blurring the road and oncoming traffic.

I tried to stuff my emotions down and prayed silently to God, "I love my family. I'm not ready to leave them. God, please give me strength to fight this cancer."

21

Those were the words that became my daily prayer, and they allowed me to sleep very well that night.

Tuesday, November 8, 2005

When I woke on Tuesday, I felt as if I had a clearly defined mission. I was going to beat cancer come hell or high water. There was no other option. I spent the entire day on the phone "working" to organize appointments and schedule my remaining tests. I called family members to report my diagnosis but decided not to call my parents quite yet. They had recently lost a close friend to cancer, and that was enough to process without throwing their daughter's battle into the mix. I also wanted to garner more information, so I would be ready to answer as many of their questions as possible.

Tuesday night, I went to bed feeling satisfied with my impending win and had no trouble falling asleep. At 10:30 p.m., I was shocked awake by my convulsing body. It shook uncontrollably as I tried to catch a deep breath, but the air stopped just short of my lungs. I had no idea what was happening. It felt as if I was going to suffocate. My first thought was that the cancer had spread to my lungs. I jostled Ron and told him to call Suzannah, but when she didn't answer, he joined my terrified state. My mind was a mess, and so my body took over. It didn't occur to either of us to take me to the emergency room. We were both overwhelmed by the previous week's events and apparently couldn't even think about making a midnight visit to the hospital. I walked the halls, went to the bathroom multiple times and grew extremely cold, shivering uncontrollably. I bundled up and tried to sleep, but it was elusive.

The night was long and fraught with bout after bout of shaking and difficulty breathing. So, when the first rays of sun finally broke through the darkness, I shot out of bed still quivering, sick and struggling for breath; but the sun was out, and that was good news. Grabbing a deep breath and straightening up, I sang the Beatles tune "Here Comes The Sun" quietly to myself while standing by my bedroom window. I had always believed that no matter how bleak my outlook, another day would always come. So, I white-knuckled that thought and stood in the diffused sunlight streaming through my window.

Moments later Suzannah called apologizing for sleeping through our call, and I felt stronger just hearing her voice. When I reported the night's events, she schooled me on anxiety attacks. It was new to me, and none of my doctors had briefed me on them, presumably because I hadn't had one and they didn't want to bring one on through the power of suggestion.

"It's really common for cancer patients to suffer anxiety attacks throughout their struggle, but there's a very easy way to knock them back. Ask your doctor to write a prescription for Lorazapam. It will act quickly and doesn't seem to have any long-term side effects," Suzannah said once again directing my care long-distance.

I hung up the phone, turned to Ron and said, "I can go to my appointments alone today. I feel so much better. Suzannah explained what was going on, and I don't feel at all scared anymore."

Ron's face twisted up in a confused look. It only took a second for me to realize how ridiculous I sounded. No doubt, that poor judgement was brought on by sleep deprivation. I was trying to minimize how much of a burden I was shouldering, but it proved to be impossible. My burden was my family's burden, and there was no way around it.

Ron and I dropped the girls off with his folks and made our way to the office of Dr. Doering, the "breast guy" and my new vascular surgeon. He was the one who saw the majority of breast cancer patients in our area, and his peers reassured me that he was the only one they would send their mothers, wives and daughters to. In his waiting room, I fidgeted nervously until the nurse came out to say that Dr. Doering was running late. Her benign words caused mild anxiety to reappear. My eyes widened, and I practiced breathing deeply as I stared at the tropical fish tank on the opposite side of the room. I searched for some peace in the fluid movement of the fish, but all I could think about was how they would be so much prettier in the open ocean, and I was as trapped and out of control as they were.

When the nurse reappeared and called my name, my relief was instant. She walked me back to an exam room with Dr. Doering following close on my heels. He had a kind and diffusing demeanor, saying very little as he performed my physical exam. When he was done, he quietly and calmly told me he would perform the lumpectomy as soon as an operating room was available. He didn't believe I had IBC and wanted to alleviate my stress as quickly as possible. I laughed out loud, unable to contain my joy.

Looking into his confident eyes, I was overcome with relief. I slumped on the exam table with a wide grin but was too exhausted to sit up straight while I listened to him organize the lumpectomy for the following Monday. He moved me to the room across the hall where there was a small tray with a familiar-looking tiny needle holding Lidocaine adjacent to a tube-shaped tool with a circular metal piece at the end that served as a knife of sorts. He

23

directed me to sit back on the exam table next to the tray and deadened my skin with the lidocaine. Next, he placed the cylindrical tool over the red area on my breast and twisted as he pushed it down, hence the name "punch biopsy." I felt the pressure, but gratefully no pain. He pulled the tool up and unloaded its contents in a liquid filled test tube. Dr. Doering dabbed the blood and affixed a bandage over the wound.

"Now, I need you to stay for a series of tests that will qualify you for surgery on Monday. Take these with you," Dr. Doering gently commanded.

He loaded me up with a fistful of orders for blood work, a urinalysis, an EKG, x-rays and a breast MRI, which would help detect if and where the tumor was spreading. I had no choice but to stay at the clinic all day if I was to be quickly cleared for surgery. His nurse escorted Ron and me to a very small room that barely passed for anything more than a box, holding one small round table and four chairs. She directed us to sit and placed a large binder on the table in front of us. Smiling softly, she proceeded to walk us through "The Binder" given to every cancer patient in an effort to help inform the person about the treatment process and keep us organized. Unfortunately, it also ushered in the stigma of having cancer, and I've never met any cancer patients who didn't grit their teeth in disdain when they talked about "The Binder." When our orientation had concluded, Ron was left in the waiting room, and I was ushered throughout the building for one test after another. Before long there was just one left, and it was a doozy. I was led into the breast MRI room, which mostly looked like all the others except that the table I was to lie on had two squares punched out of it where my chest would be. I sat on the edge of the table, and another nurse introduced herself before inserting an IV needle into my arm. She explained that during the 45-minute scan a mechanical pump would inject dye through that IV for the purpose of uncovering cancer lurking in the dark reaches of my breast tissue. I was to lie on my stomach, arms stretched out in front of me as if I was some sort of superhero. I smirked at the thought, embracing the humor in it all. She gave me earplugs to drown out the sound of the loudly knocking machine, which I later came to appreciate for its distracting qualities. Then she left the room as the machine rolled me into its mouth.

Just as I drifted off to sleep, a voice hit my ears through the magnetic machine's speakers, "You're all done!"

The moveable table was rolled back out of the MRI, and I was greeted by the nurse who had anticipated I would be a little disoriented. She helped me sit up, pulled the needle out and I was free to go. Just like that.

It was an exhausting day, but at home, I felt recharged. I was happy to have my little family around me. We still had not told the girls what was going on, but EmmaGrace was clearly growing suspicious. She confronted me after dinner demanding to know what was wrong. She had noticed how red my eyes and face were from crying, so answering with nothing wasn't going to cut it. I didn't have the energy to sit up straight, chase her around the kitchen island or have a tickle fight, burning up her last bits of energy before bed. To her it was so obvious something was wrong. Even though she was only seven years old, she wasn't buying any of my diversionary lies. So, as I gathered my words ready to spill the beans, I couldn't help but notice how bright she shined. I looked into her eyes and knew I could beat cancer, so what was the point in telling her. I decided to shift gears and casually lied to her, explaining that I just had a bad cold. It was all I could give her at that moment without spoiling her innocence so early in life. She narrowed her eyes and curled up her lip. She knew it wasn't true but just couldn't put her finger on what it was. I turned away feeling guilty about shutting her out.

Later that night, I decided to let my parents in on my diagnosis. I knew I really should have done it in person, but I told myself that there was no time to waste with the process moving so quickly. Of course, in truth, I was really just a coward. I called because I couldn't look into their eyes and see their devastation after hearing that their baby was hosting cancer. Today, I have no recollection of that conversation and can't even say if they responded before I hung up, but I wrote about it in my journals, which became a surrogate memory during that period in my life. Ironically, what was memorable was needing a hug from them when I hung up, and I'm sure they needed one just as much as I did. As I lay in bed that night, I fell asleep thinking about my girls. EmmaGrace was so lively and perceptive. Hannah was so strong and confident. She didn't talk very much, but when I looked into her eyes, I swore I heard her saying, "It's going to be my way, and I say you're going to be OK, Mommy." Drawing from the admiration I had for my beautiful girls, my strength took hold again. I was so blessed to have them. I knew that whatever cancer I had, it was in for one hell of a fight.

Wednesday, November 9, 2005
The next day was a relatively normal day. EmmaGrace went to school, and I called the principal to tell her my story. I stuffed my fear down deep and displayed only confidence as I asked her to watch over EmmaGrace who had not yet been told what was happening but knew something was up. We planned to tell her over the weekend, and I wanted the school to be ready to handle whatever emotions she showed up with on Monday. After we hung up, the principal notified EmmaGrace's second grade teacher and another teacher

who had beaten breast cancer five years earlier. They put a book in my daughter's backpack that was written to help kids with a parent's diagnosis and a note of encouragement to me. I swelled with gratitude, and by the evening, I felt stronger yet and ready to win. I measured out the tumor on a ruler, sure that something so tiny would never take me down.

Friday, November 11, 2005
Unfortunately, as it goes with the roller coaster ride of cancer, my positive attitude was ripped away from me on Friday. I went to see our homeopathic pediatrician, Dr. Keating, to talk about alternative ways to support my body through this process. He had me squirming in the chair while he described injections of mistletoe into my stomach to help lessen the side-effects of chemotherapy. During his short lecture, my cell phone rang, and I thanked God. It was Dr. Doering. Ron, uncharacteristically impatient, had contacted him demanding the results of my skin biopsy and breast MRI. But with the words that were about to follow, I would've rather heard more about needles and liquid mistletoe.

Sitting in the chair facing Dr. Keating, I heard Dr. Doering say, "It's not good news. The tumor appears to be approaching five centimeters, and the skin biopsy confirmed it to be inflammatory breast cancer. I am so sorry. I was wrong, and I've set up an appointment for you with the best oncologist around. You'll see Dr. Harper at 3:00 p.m. I'll still see you on Monday, but I will insert your mediport instead, and you'll be starting chemo on Tuesday."

Just like that.

My head was spinning in a cyclone of test results and emotions. The tears were pouring unchecked out of my eyes. I sat in the chair not saying anything, just crying. Dr. Keating sat quietly, just waiting. When I pulled myself together, I thanked him and took out my list of errands to run before I picked up Hannah from day care. The absolute urgency to stock up on wipes, diapers and toilet paper in advance of the impending storm tmade me stumble out of his office like a zombie running towards the living shopping across the street at Target.

I blundered through the aisles in a quagmire of panic, searching my being for any tiny seed of sense. I was completely in my own head space, and nothing else existed until I collided with a friend in the toilet paper aisle. All smiles, she asked how I was, which generally was a throw away question, socially speaking. She didn't wait for my response before recounting the latest developments in her husband's campaign for judge and the unfortunate revelation of a once sordid affair, but I was thankful for her lack of pause, excusing me from responding and leaving my thoughts bogged down in a thick marsh fog like a scene from *The Hounds Of Baskerville*. I slogged through the muck, snatching a small smile and a shred of a laugh. I told her good luck and, without toilet paper, headed for the checkout counter with diapers and wipes in hand. In slow motion I raced to the car entirely aware of the chaotic firing of each synapse. How did a smallish tumor morph into something so horrible? The breast MRI showed a whopping pyramid-shaped tumor, lacing itself through my dermis in search of the dermal lymphatics, its gateway to the largest organ in the body – my skin. From there IBC could enter my main lymph system, creating a sanctuary to block my natural cleansing system and overtake my body like a tsunami.

The pathology lab report for my skin punch biopsy stated, "Sections of the punch biopsy show small nests of infiltrating carcinoma in the mid to deep dermis. The cells are arranged in solid nests and cords and exhibit nuclear pleomorphism with prominent nucleoli. No dermal lymphocytic involvement is identified."

From that small sample of my skin, it appeared that the cancer hadn't reached my dermal lymphatics, and that was huge, but I was painfully aware that another section of my skin might've told a different story. I held onto the hope that because of Suzannah, the cancer had been caught earlier than usual. While my symptoms had not been familiar to the doctors in our area, I had Suzannah, who was well aware of them. She had gained invaluable experience at Sloan-Kettering and knew what a simple red spot on the surface of the breast could mean. Most descriptions of IBC on the Internet and at the doctor's office described a breast red, inflamed, warm to the touch, and having the texture of an orange peel. In actuality if it had reached that point, it would've been moving like the *Loony Tunes'* tasmanian devil through my body, leaving me little hope to survive.

Hosting IBC was absolutely surreal. I had invested myself so fully in having a lesser, beatable cancer and called Suzannah before driving to the oncologist's office. My first question was her number one dreaded question.

"What are my chances of survival?" I asked.

She refused to discuss it with me and responded very plainly, "Survival rates are not important. You are either 0% or 100%. Every person is different. Frankly, you are not a statistic. You are you, and you'll do whatever you have to do to be 100%. I would suggest you stay off the Internet."

I could barely see through my tears. The road was a blur as I drove to Dr. Harper's office where Ron was already waiting. After parking the car at the Regional Cancer Center, I became suddenly aware that the healing had already begun. During my call to Suzannah, she gave me the IBC treatment protocol Sloan-Kettering was successfully using, and I wrote everything in a notebook, which became my designated cancer notebook. It was a sacred item for me throughout my treatment. It wasn't "The Binder;" it was "my" book. It was where I kept all of my doctor's cell phone numbers, the types and quantities of drugs I was being given, lists of what to do and where to be, names of people who were a part of my growing team, questions I had for my doctors, updates from my many doctor visits, and procedures and tests, but perhaps equally as important was what I kept in the back. The back pages were dedicated to the list of people I needed to thank. Each time someone made us a meal, sent me flowers, made me a piece of jewelry, took me to lunch, or made any other kind gesture, I wrote a thank you note. Doing that really helped me to understand that I wasn't alone, and without that notebook I would've lost track of the huge network supporting my recovery.

In the exam room at the cancer center Ron and I listened to Dr. Harper's thoughts; and as soon as he took a pause, I launched into the instructions Suzannah had given me. His plan was different from what she had laid out. So, like the other doctors, he listened to what I had to say. His empathetic calm diffused my anxiety, and I was heartened by the genuine connection he made with me. When I was done, he closed his computer and pulled out his cell phone.

"Let me call her right now," Dr. Harper said.

I was stunned but dutifully gave him her number. They talked for the better part of my appointment and agreed to work together over the weekend on my customized protocol to ensure chemo started on Tuesday. After he hung up with Suzannah, he turned to me and asked if I had experienced any anxiety.

"Yes! That's right! I was supposed to tell you that. I've had bouts of shaking and problems breathing with rapid-fire bowel elimination," I exclaimed with an inappropriately placed moment of exuberance.

Years before I had something similar when a bear terrorized our campsite in the middle of the night. It was a very mild anxiety attack by comparison and ended as soon as we were able to sneak into the canoe and push it off shore. The cancer-related anxiety attacks were far worse, surprising me when I least expected it and seeming to have nothing to do with my emotional state but naming them afforded me a small modicum of comfort. It took the unfamiliar,

28

diffused it and made it familiar, providing me some control over it. Dr. Harper bolstered my control by adding Lorazapam, a drug designed to almost immediately take the anxiety level down. That little white pill was like magic for me. It would've been such a useful service to cancer patients and their families if clinics were allowed to offer it in a gumball-type machine at the door. Instead of the slip of paper from a prescription pad, maybe one day they will hand patients a gift card to swipe in a vending machine, spilling those tiny little helpers into our needy little hands before leaving the clinic. It was the one prescription drug I struggled to let go of, and not because it was addictive, but because the anxiety of recurrence never really went away. Even so, nine years after that first diagnosis, I was finally brave enough to say good-bye to that calming little crutch.

Before leaving the cancer center on that first visit, I paused at the door and asked Dr. Harper one more critical question.

"What is my chance of survival?"

He refused to answer it directly. He said something along the lines of, "Let's see how it goes.

Armed with "The Binder" and my notebook, Ron and I left the cancer center that first day silently wading through the lingering shock. During our meeting I took a multitude of notes, which afforded me some level of detached focus. The notebook kept me engaged. Without it my mind would've been floating out in space and not at all advocating for my life. Ron was not great at processing on the spot. My brain was on rapid fire while his was still working through the implications of a wife that would likely die and two young children that would be left motherless. For me Suzannah and Dr. Harper provided a sort of calm or maybe just resolve. I was doing what I could, and there wasn't anything more for me to do on that day except fill the prescription and pop that pill.

Over the weekend, Suzannah lobbed the ball back to her caché of doctors in New York. I had no involvement in the conversations, and it was the first of many times throughout my treatment that I had to relinquish control, have faith and trust the professionals. Over the weekend, emails flew between Suzannah, my oncologist and her doctors at Sloan Kettering as they hatched my treatment plan to be cracked wide open on Monday. Meanwhile, amid anxiety attacks and blubbering breakdowns, I tried to hold the words of Dr. Tousignant in the forefront of my mind, "Treat it like job."

29

If having cancer was a job, I needed more detail on what I was up against, which meant scouring the Internet for every little bit of information I could find. Unfortunately, what I found was a very little bit of information. Since the cancer I had was so rare, pretty much every site carried the same description, and the first piece of information that jumped out was that thousands of women were diagnosed each year with IBC, a little known but extremely deadly form of breast cancer. It was more difficult to detect because it didn't present as a lump like most breast cancers. IBC cells spread out in "nests" or sheets, so a lump was rarely felt or seen on a mammogram. Each site offered me the same dismal prognosis. IBC had one of the lowest survival rates of the breast cancers and was often misdiagnosed as an infection. While the doctors and patients waited for antibiotics to work, the cancer quickly crept into the lymph system mounting a complete takeover of the woman's body. That process could take as little as a few weeks or as much as a few months, and it almost didn't matter what stage it was because the survival rates were all bleak. I had stage IV, although I hadn't yet been told, and that gave me an 11% chance of survival after five years as compared to other invasive breast cancers which were at 87%. The average survival rate period for my diagnosis was just 21 months.

After I read those statistics, I fully expected anxiety to well up again, but it didn't. Instead, I had a job to do, and I felt the strength inside me grow. It was utterly impossible that I would die. My girls were just babies aged two and seven, and I wasn't going to leave them motherless. I just wasn't. It was time to get my head right and build a strategy for my success.

Saturday, November 12, 2005
The Saturday before I was to start chemo was a wonderfully windy fall day. We took a family hike on the trails meandering throughout our farm's 60 acres, which was something we did often. Ron loved bonfires and had created several fire pits along the trail, giving each one its own name reflective of the terrain it was located in. On that day, we found comfort in the "Secret Woods." EmmaGrace loved being the older sister and took Hannah's stroller from me, leaning into it as she pushed it down the rutted trails. When the trail got rough, worn from heavy rains, her eyes narrowed, and her tenacity took hold as she threw all of her strength into the handle, heaving it over the rocky obstacles. A couple of times EmmaGrace had to ask Hannah to get out and walk but forgot to adjust her thrust and sent the empty stroller sailing over the rugged terrain, crashing into the tall grass lining the trail. We all laughed so hard we cried.

Before we arrived at the woods, I needed just one more delay. I desperately

30

wanted to take advantage of the blustering winds and fly our kites in the open, tall grass prairie I had restored six years before. The girls laughed wildly, following the dips, dives and crashes of their kites, loving the chaotic, twisting movements as they sailed in unpredictable patterns over the prairie. As soon as I was joyfully lost in their unbridled thrill, the memory of what was to come next slapped me hard on the cheek. My smile dropped abruptly, but not wanting them to see it, I plastered it back on, hoping they wouldn't recognize my insincerity.

Finally exhausted by the chase, we made our way to the "Secret Woods." I settled Hannah into her stroller for a little nap, tightly tucking a fleece blanket around her and then closing the attached plastic cover to help keep the warmth in. Sensing something was coming, EmmaGrace stared at me with a focus I had never seen from her. She was piercing the depth of my soul, searching for a preview of what was to come. Ron also had a look I had never seen. The pain and fear in his eyes scared me. I felt a burst of adrenaline release in me and restrained myself from running back to the house. I had no idea how to comfort him, let alone her, and wasn't I the one who needed comforting after all? I sapped all of my energy stores, trying to come up with the right words for my seven-year-old daughter and had nothing left for him.

Ron got the fire going, and we all let the warmth wash over our hands and faces. I looked into EmmaGrace's beseeching green eyes and then down to the pine needles littered on the ground. Fighting to drag my eyes back to hers, I explained that I had cancer. It was crazy to hear those words coming out of my mouth. How could I possibly describe cancer to a seven-year-old?

The best I could do was to say, "Honey, I have some very sick cells in my body, and when they got sick, they changed. Instead of working with me, they are fighting against me. They're called cancer, and it's time for me to get them out."

EmmaGrace stared at me in silence, but I could see her gears turning.

"I don't want you to worry. You know Mama is strong even though it will look as if I'm not. The medicine they're going to give me will make me very tired, and it will seem as if I have a really bad stomach flu during the battle, but I'm really going to be fighting to beat the cancer," I concluded.

Having already read the book her school had given to us, Ron and I hoped we were armed with the answers EmmaGrace needed to hear. Luckily for us, she jumped right into the first question they covered, "Can I catch

31

cancer?" Ron perked up and with a slight knowing smile gave me a nod as if to say, "I've got this."

He immediately paraphrased from the book, "Cancer is like a broken arm in that you can't catch a broken arm from someone, and you can't catch cancer either."

She was relieved and scared. With me at the doctors all the time, it had been a very hard week for her. Sadly, we had made it even harder by keeping her in the dark when clearly something serious was happening. In hindsight we should've told her sooner. Then, we all would've been in the same boat, and she wouldn't have felt so isolated. The usually impulsive EmmaGrace took a minute to think about what Ron had said.

She, like her dad, pronounced, "Well, don't worry, Mama. I'll help you."

I cast that beam of uncontrollable love light her way and knew instantly I would absolutely be as formidable as my foe.

Back at the house, Ron put Hannah down for a deeper nap and then read EmmaGrace the cancer book while I listened horizontal on the pea green, antique couch. She got a giggle out of the fact that her question was the same as the girl in the book and both daddies had answered it in the same way. I chuckled at the funny "coincidence" before discussing what was to come for me.

"I'm going to lose my hair, Honey, and have to start wearing a wig or hat," I said nervously.

Unfazed, EmmaGrace gave me a big bear hug and said, "I love hats! You made the right choice by going to the doctor, Mama! I'm very proud of you."

The next day, my sweet little second grader, who was itching to do something for me, "took" me hat shopping after breakfast. We tried on every single hat, tucking my long hair up under it to see what I would look like bald; then, we'd laugh, having no idea what it would mean for me to actually be bald. In the end she picked out five hats for me, and a cheetah hat with matching gloves for herself.

Back at home EmmaGrace asked, "Mama, can I fix your hair before it falls out?"

Tears formed in my eyes. "Of course," I said, knowing that it would be the last time for a long time that I would have the privilege of being my daughter's hair doll.

I was completely in the dark about how profound a moment that was. It was unknowable how devastated we would all be by the loss of something seemingly so unimportant as my hair.

Monday, November 14, 2005
Monday morning was met with a call from my oncologist, Dr. Harper. He was calling to let me know that he and the doctors at Memorial Sloan-Kettering had developed a plan, and it had already been set in motion.

"I would've never done it this way, but it makes perfect sense," he assured me. "Together, we'll deliver cutting-edge treatment to not only you, but other Wisconsin women diagnosed with IBC."

I allowed myself a moment to feel proud, hoping someone else would benefit from my experience, and nearly one year later, someone did. My family doctor told me that because of my case, she was able to give an early diagnosis to one of her other patients. I felt deeply relieved for a woman I would probably never meet but didn't allow myself to think about her potential situation. It was enough to know she was getting an added advantage against her cancer.

Dr. Harper's call set my nerves jumping in anticipation for the surgery scheduled later that afternoon. Dr. Doering would thread a catheter through one of my veins and attach it semi-permanently to a half-dollar-sized silicone bladder stitched in place just under my skin. The thought of it made me shudder. I'm not sure why. I've had a number of other surgeries over the years and even had screws put in my knee, but somehow the mediport bulging out from under my skin just below my collarbone was different. It was a symbol that would be hard to hide. Why I felt I needed to hide it is anyone's guess. I suppose I saw it as a billboard advertising my private battle. At 11:30 a.m., we left for the hospital, and Ron seemed relieved. He was a doer, and we were about to start doing. In the surgical ward, he handed me off to the nurse who prepped me for surgery; then, he let out an audible sigh of relief as he faded into the wallpaper. The nurses bustled around me as they inserted the intravenous needle into my vein, took my vitals, slipped hospital booties on my feet and infused valium into my IV before whisking me away. It was a little like being a football handed off from one player to the next with the last pass going to Dr. Doering for the

33

touchdown! I was out. My mediport was inserted, and I was home by 6:30 p.m. Just like that.

Managing our little family to accommodate my needs had become a team event. On the day of my surgery, Ron's parents picked up EmmaGrace after school and kept her overnight. My parents picked Hannah up from day care and brought her home to sleep in her own bed. When we walked in the door, I saw my dad first. He looked so scared and completely devastated by my fragile appearance. Doing something was helpful for him, but seeing me brought tears to his eyes. I felt myself going to that familiar role of pushing my own feelings of needy fragility aside, digging deep for strength so I could try to help them feel better. I had no idea how to comfort them other than to put a smile on my face and echo Ron's words that I would be fine. I didn't want them to see the suffering I felt and just couldn't imagine being in their shoes.

With Ron it was different. Our conversations had become generally uncomfortable with me either looking down or off to the side, and always careful not to meet his eyes for fear I would get sucked into his dread that I would die. I prayed constantly that he would believe in me but ultimately knew that I was the only one who needed to believe. When I started to crumble, I repeated my mantras or created a new one to serve the situation. I mentally repeated, "Lord, allow me to be stronger than my foe" and prayed my girls would not know life without a mother. Where everyone else saw a battle lost, I visualized a long road to successfully traverse. I kept the win at the forefront of my mind and fell asleep assisted by the lingering effects of anesthesia.

Tuesday, November 15, 2005
The next day was my first chemo day. I woke up a little sore from the surgery, but I was ready. The fight was on. Dr. Doering had left a catheter in place to make that first day easier. The tiny plastic tube was attached to a shut off valve, which kept my blood from dripping out of my body. The whole apparatus was taped to my chest over the incision bandage, which kept it from catching on my clothes. Gratefully, Dr. Doering had thought to spare me the poke when I had my blood drawn and the chemo delivered. In the future to get that same benefit, I would apply the Emla Cream given to me by the cancer center. It was essentially Lidocaine formulated to deaden the pain before each subsequent poke. Ron dropped me off at the cancer center and took Hannah to his parents' home. It felt strange sitting in that waiting room alone. I felt completely out of place among the other patients. I had all of my hair, and they didn't. I was at least 20 years younger than the

youngest person there. I awkwardly smiled at each of them not knowing what was appropriate behavior in a cancer treatment waiting room. It was a new subculture for me, and one that was sadly growing to become more of the norm. I decided not to engage any further and engrossed myself in the reading materials left on the coffee table. I picked up a pamphlet bearing the title of a now defunct breast cancer organization called *Y ME?* At the sight of that simple question, anger percolated up from my depths.

Luckily, I couldn't wallow too long in those feelings before Lynne walked over, gave me a big smile, and said, "We're ready for you."

There was no turning back. I had officially climbed aboard the cancer train, and the first stop was the lab. Nurse Lynn had a wonderfully cheery demeanor, making it easy for me to trust that I was in good hands. She was a foot or so shorter than me, and her turned up face was round and rosy as she beckoned me to follow her through the lobby. I found it hard to believe that she could ever frown and followed obediently, staying two steps behind, and completely subservient to her elevated state of joy. At the blood draw room, Lynn directed me to sit in a brown recliner placed in the corner of the room.

She pointed to the chair with enthusiasm and said, "This is yours today!"

When she saw the conspicuous catheter extending out from the quarter-sized silicon bladder sitting just under my skin, she let out a giddy laugh.

"Isn't Dr. Doering awesome?" she asked not waiting for my reply.

His consideration had made the day pain-free for me and a breeze for her. I smiled through pursed lips and watched as she brought a tray of vials over to the small table next to my chair. She inserted the needle into the catheter and then turned the plastic winged switch to open the flow. I watched the clear plastic tube change to red as my blood raced through the line and into the first vial. Lynn closed the valve, picked up another one and repeated the process. That first blood draw was my baseline. It was the one all future results would be measured against. I was at ground zero, and as far as I was concerned, there was nowhere to go but up. With no pain, I relaxed into chit chat until she was done and then followed her to the chemotherapy treatment room.

At the door Lynn motioned me to step inside, but my feet were firmly planted at the threshold. I was unable to move even as my chemo nurse, Denise, slid past me into "the room." It was another hand off. From the doorway I saw an oversized brown reclining chair sitting next to a gurney-type bed. The metal posts for hanging IV bags between the chair and the gurney were nothing different than what I had seen during my knee surgeries, but somehow the IV bags had a more sinister look against the backdrop of cancer. There was a small grey counter with a lower counter attached and a wheeled stool underneath it to provide a temporary desk for the oncologist. I fought the urge to bolt as my mind worked fast, running through the potential scenarios if I had. Fortunately, reason won out, and I concluded nothing good would come of it. Somewhat defeated, I committed and took a seat in one of the corner chairs meant for family members, not yet ready to take my rightful place in the chemo chair. A flash of my dead body on the gurney popped into my mind just as Ron rushed into the room like a kid late to class.

Denise paused negligibly when I sat in the wrong chair and then pleasantly began "chemo day." She took my vitals, explained that I would be hooked up to the IVs through which two different chemotherapies would be pumped for nearly seven hours. There was something about Benadryl to avert an allergic reaction and steroids to help my body accept the chemo. Steroids would also serve to stimulate my appetite to help keep me from dying of malnutrition. Somewhere between 20-40% of cancer patients die from malnutrition, and I wasn't going to be one of them. So, I promised myself I would eat. I tried to listen to Denise, but my mind wouldn't stop bouncing to the only question I wanted answered. I just had to stop her.

"What are my odds of surviving?" I forcefully asked, wanting to know if going through chemo would even make a difference.

Without much of a pause, Denise answered, "There are a lot of people in here buying time."

Just like that. It was the answer I had been waiting for. She gave it to me straight. She had done exactly what I had hoped, but surprisingly, I couldn't take it. I wouldn't take it. I needed positive, hopeful people around me each and every day. Even though I liked Denise, I couldn't handle her brutal honesty. She and I were slated to spend a ton of time together, and I needed her to believe I would make it because despite the grim statistics, I had already decided I would. I knew my medical team was mostly going through the motions for me, but I needed my nurse not to let on, so I asked for someone else to work with me at my next appointment.

When Denise left the room to tell Dr. Harper that I was ready, I deliberately decided to fix my attitude. I needed to be happy and positive, which surely would be a key part of my healing. All of the literature in "The Binder" said so. I looked over to Ron who had a water bottle with him mixed with the black walnut tincture we had concocted from our trees in the backyard. The dirty yellow-colored water was purported to be anti-bacterial, anti-fungal and anti-viral. Anti-cancer wasn't on that list, but it should've been. It was exactly what I needed. I took his bottle and placed it strategically on the desk where Dr. Harper would have to move it in order to put his computer down. Then, I sat back laughing to myself while Ron looked at me questioningly.

I chuckled and said, "Just wait."

I heard one of the hard plastic flags outside the door hit the wall. The oncologist had put it back in line to let the nurse know he was inside. He opened the door and grinned widely at me. His nurse, Mary, gave a cordial hello as she slipped past him to assume her position at the window.

Standing in front of me, gazing down with kind eyes, he asked, "Hello, how are you today?"

"I don't know," I dutifully responded trying not to laugh.

Unfazed by my response, he smiled at Ron and turned to his desk. Dr. Harper rolled the stool out, sat down and went to place his computer on the desk as he had done 20 times each day. Absentmindedly, he picked up the bottle and turned to hand it to me. Then, he noted the color and looked at us quizzically.

I engaged his questioning expression with a straight face and asked, "This is what our water looks like at home. Do you think that's why I have cancer?"

His mouth dropped open; then, a twinkle appeared in his eye, and a broad smile moved across the doctor's face.

"Oh, so this is how it's going to be?" he goaded me.

"Yes, it is. It's the only way for me to win," I responded, recalling Norman Cousins who used humor to battle and recover from ankylosing spondylitis disease.

"Well, I can do that with you. I will enjoy doing that with you," Dr. Harper said handing the bottle back to Ron, and with his shoulders shaking slightly, turned to open his computer.

Mary looked confused by my jovial move. She knew she was supposed to laugh as well, but it was outside of the protocol box. Normally, the first chemo appointment would have been very difficult and full of dread, but somehow I wasn't acting the way everyone else did. However, once the normal conversation began, she comfortably settled back into her regular role. When I seemed satisfied and had no more questions about what was going to happen to me that day, Dr. Harper slapped the top of his notebook computer down and stood up.

"I'll let Denise know you're ready. If you need to speak to me, just let Mary know," he said with a wink and then left the room.

For a brief moment, it was just Ron and I. Neither one of us knew what to say in that awkward silence. We were in a completely new situation that felt entirely alien to us. Luckily, Denise quickly returned and asked if I preferred the bed or the chair since I was going to feel sleepy and she wanted me to be comfortable. The bed was out of the question. I wanted to sit up, watch television, read, talk and just see what was happening as if I wasn't sick at all. I fell deeply into the comfortable cushions of the chair and turned my head to the right, looking away as Denise flushed the pic line attached to my mediport with tissue plasminogen activator (TPA) to clear blood clots away. She rolled the metal pole next to my chair, placed a bag of saline onto it and then left the room. When she returned, she held a stainless-steel tray with three very large syringes filled with a disturbing red-colored fluid called Adriamyacin chemotherapy and a bag of clear liquid called Cytoxan, another chemo drug. I felt confused and a little flushed as fear moved through my cells.

Suzannah's words of wisdom flashed through me, "If you're afraid, just think how the cancer feels? You're stronger."

"As I explained, you'll be getting two kinds of chemotherapy every other week," Denise calmly reported.

"I get it, but red? I feel as if I committed some egregious crime and you're my executioner by lethal injection. Red? Couldn't they come up with something more soothing like lavender? I know that all chemos can't be clear, but who was the idiot that thought red was a good color for cancer patients?" Those words just exploded out of me.

I wasn't expecting an answer, and Denise didn't disappoint. She moved automatically through her routine, shooting me a weak smile now and again before ending with the obligatory question of "All set?" I was bound to a

38

plastic bag hanging from a metal pole. Of course I was set.

Denise collected the tray with used cotton swabs, gauze pads, discarded plastic wrappers and the rest of the medical garbage that had housed what I hoped would be my salvation before quietly switching off the light and closing the door. While I adjusted myself in the chair, I was trying to discern the mumbling voice I could hear through the door when it opened, and Debbie appeared. She was a massage therapist I had previously seen, and as she gazed down on me, a smile tempered with sadness took form on her face. Her job on Tuesdays and Thursdays was to provide massages to patients in treatment.

"I was stunned to see your name. You were so healthy. I wondered why I hadn't seen you in a while," she said. "Would you like me to give you a massage to help pass the time and relieve some anxiety?" she asked.

I didn't want to be rude, but I didn't really want a massage with a two-inch curved needle taped to my chest. I myself was moving gingerly for fear it would pull out. So, I did what any well-mannered Wisconsin girl would do. I thanked her and accepted her gift. While she worked to relieve my stress, I glanced at Ron and gritted my teeth. It was a test of endurance to make it through that 15-minute session, and when it was all over, I thanked her, neglecting to say that I was feeling much more on edge.

After the massage Ron went to work, and I sat or slept most of the day. I was alone. My parents wanted to come, but I didn't want them to see me like that. Friends also offered, but I couldn't have anyone in my space feeling sorry for me or watching me sleep, and most of all, I didn't want to feel as if I needed to entertain anyone. Instead, I spent my day internalizing the fear and focusing on being stronger than cancer. Periodically, Denise checked in on me as I dozed, and one of those times, she left behind a tray of food. I took a few sips of soup and left the rest to waste. The cloak of loneliness drooped over me as I stared blankly at the wall and began to pray. I prayed for strength. I prayed for my girls not to have to suffer the trauma of losing their mother. I prayed that I would handle the chemo well. I prayed to beat the cancer. Then, I drifted back to sleep.

Ron arrived at the end of my poisoning. It was hard to look at him. His expression was filled with doubt, or maybe it was my feelings projected on him. Either way, I turned away, trying not to fall into his vortex of fear. It seemed Ron's statements that I would be fine were just empty encouragement. He didn't believe it but didn't know what else to say. The energy of "the end" was heavy around me. While Dr. Harper did not tell me then, eight years later, he told me his plan was to just keep me comfortable until I died because he didn't expect me to make it, and even though he didn't share those words at the time, I sensed it.

Denise pulled the needle from my chest, cleaned the hole left behind, and then covered it with a bandage. She handed me a printed list of appointments that I was expected to attend throughout the rest of the week and sent me on my way. It was all very anti-climactic, very matter of fact. I was waiting to hear some sort of Woop-woop! That's one down. Way to go!

Instead, I got more instructions from Denise delivered in a matter-of-fact way, "Come back tomorrow for your Neulasta shot. It will help boost your bone marrow's ability to produce white blood cells and strengthen your immune system."

I mumbled an obligatory, "Thank you" and stumbled out to the car.

I had always been insanely busy, perpetually and simultaneously moving in multiple directions, but with the cancer diagnosis, my schedule of appointments and tests made my previous calendar look bare. Happily, my hospital also served as my personal assistant, scheduling and synching all of my appointments in blocks of time and at the same location. What used to be packed with variety had become a calendar with room for little else than eradicating cancer. No one asked what my schedule was or whether I could make the appointments they had set for me. It was simply expected that I would. That first treatment day seemed as if I had been drafted into some sort of boot camp. I had no choice in the matter and had no idea what to expect. They made the rules, and if I had any hope of surviving, I would follow them to a tee.

Slumped over and deflated, I walked out to the car as my self-esteem drained from every pore on my body. I was afraid to be noticed, wanting to stop the process and go back to normal, but my normal had been left behind forever. There was no going back. By the time we got home, my mental state had already started to recover. I discovered there was truly nothing that boosted my spirit more than leaving the catacombs of the cancer center and being injected with a little fresh air. The mother in me rallied to help EmmaGrace with her homework while Ron made dinner. After dinner I read *The Hope Tree* and *Three Brave Women* to the girls before tucking them into bed. They were so innocent and sweet. I couldn't begin to imagine what they were doing with the information we shared about a nasty-colored poison being put in my body to kill cancer.

Wednesday, November 16, 2005

It was a new day. I woke up feeling great. I took EmmaGrace to school and decided I was going to do just fine on chemo. I was strong and expected to stay that way. Denise had said that how I responded to chemo that first time would be a strong indicator of how I would respond throughout. While that was a positive notion on her part, it wouldn't be long before I discovered that she was entirely wrong.

At school EmmaGrace beamed, expressing how proud she was of me. For her it was the coolest thing that I had been poisoned to get better. What's more, I was happy and at school with her the very next day. To her I was some sort of a wonder woman – a definite superhero. At her second grade classroom, she dropped my hand, leaving me at the door.

She ran in and proudly shouted, "My mom was poisoned yesterday, and she's still here!"

Uh-oh! I could just hear the parents at that small private school freaking out. Mr. Yuck would be a farce. All cleaning cupboards and first aid cabinets would be fair game.

Her teacher and I jumped in, "That's not exactly the way it was!"

We looked at each other with a chuckle. We had actually said the same thing at the same time. I wanted to shout "Jinx," but EmmaGrace yelled it first.

Then, she followed it with, "Mom, you have to say pickles before Mrs. Walberg does!"

It was the new antidote to the old jinx.

"Pickles. So, what EmmaGrace means," I continued, "is that I had to have some medicine yesterday that looked just like poison. Who likes to take medicine?" I asked with a disgusted scrunched up smile.

The kids twisted their faces and spit out, "Yuck."

Crises averted. EmmaGrace's teacher and I walked her out into the hall and explained that she wouldn't be able to share everything that went on at home with her classmates, and I knew that was going to be even tougher for her than having a mom with cancer. From behind me I heard a warm hello and turned to find Marge. She was the kindergarten teacher who was five years out from a breast cancer diagnosis. Gratefully, she had volunteered

41

to be EmmaGrace's ears at school, offering to give my daughter her full attention during recess. What a gift! I made a deal with EmmaGrace that she could tell Marge anything she wanted to but would have to keep her classmates in the dark. She agreed.

My next stop was the cancer center for the first bi-weekly immune booster shot, Neulasta. In some ways, that little shot in my fanny proved to be harder than the chemo. It was designed to protect patients by boosting their production of white blood cells in the bone marrow, strengthening the body's immune response. However, the following morning, I woke up with intense pain in my sternum, legs, arms and hips; in fact, every joint in my nearly six-foot frame ached. My long bones felt deeply bruised, and the suffering was compounded by the delayed effects of chemo. It was hard to believe that Neulasta and chemotherapy were working for me. I was overwhelmed by nausea and grabbed for Decadron, one of the anti-nausea medications in my cancer center bag of tricks. It made my eyes jump, causing dizziness, which made the race to the bathroom chaotic every time I had to throw up. I reached into my bag and pulled out two more prescriptions, searched my few cryptic notes for some helpful instruction, and finding none, desperately popped a Compazine followed by a Lorazepam; the result was nothing good. Crushed, my misery deepened as I sank into the pea green couch, curling up under the afghan my mom had crocheted for me.

Friday wasn't much better. Having been up most of the night, I was exhausted and unable to think clearly. Before Hannah got up, Ron gave me a glass of grape juice, which was promptly ejected from my stomach. He quickly pulled out "The Binder" and gathered together some other foods I might be able to eat. I managed to get a little yogurt down with a couple of saltines. A few bites of a peanut butter bagel went down hard with a chaser of milk and chamomile tea. I grazed at the mini buffet Ron laid out, taking tiny nibbles of each food until I felt the reflux swell from the depths. In the end, all of our efforts were futile. Nothing stayed down. Debilitated by the exertion, I collapsed on the couch and dozed.

It was Hannah's day to be home with me, so Ron organized her breakfast and left her to play before disappearing into his basement office, working to earn some money so we could pay our already mounting medical bills. I wanted to "be a trooper," but I had my doubts. Luckily, as most things go, it worked out just fine. I mostly watched her twirl, sing and play with her dolls from the sideways vantage point of my head on the couch. Usually, I felt joy blanket me as her wide grin flashed with each spin, but after chemo number one, I blankly stared at her for about two hours before calling Ron for reinforcements. My two-year-old's sounds were so amplified in my head that they became overwhelming to endure. I hated the feeling of helplessness and weakness. All I had done that day was lay on the couch, forcing a smile now and again, but it was exhausting. Never loving to nap, I found myself stressed by how terrible I felt, and instead of playing with my happy little two-year-old, I was in bed developing a crushing headache. Somewhere in that self-pity, I managed to doze ever so briefly, waking just as Hannah went down for her nap. Ron left to pick up EmmaGrace from school, and I emerged from my room seeking out a glass of cranberry juice.

Normally quite chatty, I had started to ration my words, which resulted in very little conversation between Ron and me. Normally fairly quiet, Ron got quieter as he took on being mom, dad, breadwinner and caretaker. That was a tough gig made even more difficult by the fact that our farm was 25 minutes away from school and even further from family. We were in the boonies, so finding help with the kids meant leaving them far from home, which I hated. I wanted my family close. I needed them close. So, Ron drove... a lot.

Thursday, November 17, 2005
The siege was on. The war was waged. My arsenal was stocked. I was a warrior, but that sounded a little like Robert Bly's *Iron Warrior: A Book About Men*. I planned to become the victor and one day see myself as the cancer annihilator. I wondered why references to cancer were generally war related because, honestly, I felt more put upon than at war. I was a civilian trapped in a war zone, not a soldier that had enlisted to fight. Maybe I was more like the victim of a mugging. I wasn't brave. I was dealing with a disease that was thrust upon me, and being called a survivor felt weak. The more I judged the widely accepted terminology of my disease, the more embarrassed I felt not to embrace it. Was I a traitor? Was I fighting a war or planning my recovery? I supposed it was a win to beat cancer, but what would the spoils of the war be? As the years progressed, the first round of spoils weren't worth the paper they were written on. I worked hard to recover, rebuilding a body assaulted by the toxic tools of the trade. The side-effects of treatment and the subsequent treatment of the side-effects were all I had to show for my labor. The battle was mine alone. Everyone processes the medications differently, and by all counts, I was a drug weakling. Living with them and their "benefit" was like living in a war-torn city each day, picking through rubble for scraps of food. It would take years for me to get back to some semblance of normal, and it would obviously never really look the same.

The impact of cancer treatment hit me hard and fast. Exactly 21 days after my "shower of discovery," I was in the throes of contamination even The Toxic Avenger would run from. I felt as if I was in an exorcism that would last at least a year, and like a broken record, I prayed for strength.

I imagined God saying, "Yes, I got it. You want to live. You don't need to keep repeating it. I won't forget."

The long-drawn-out attempt by chemo to purge the squatting evil would eventually cause my strength to wane and my mind to aimlessly drift towards death, making it seem that God did forget my pleas or else wasn't all that interested in my requests. Tangible strength was at best elusive. I worked to endure the agony of that first treatment. By Friday, the long morning of bathroom visits and a burning sensation in my esophagus compelled me to break the cycle and grab a task that would take me out of the house. I wondered if removing myself from those walls would help me feel any better because being cooped up and stumbling from the couch to the bathroom was a miserable way to exist. So, I slowly showered and dug deep to fill my lungs with air

"I'm going to pick EmmaGrace up from school," I told Ron, meeting his eye.

He looked at me doubtfully but didn't resist.

"Call if you can't make it," he said.

When I arrived at the school, EmmaGrace wasn't at all surprised to see me in the driver's seat. She hadn't been home to see my guts in the toilet, so to her, it was a perfectly normal day.

"I have to do a report on whales, Momma," she reported climbing into the car.

"That sounds like fun," I responded with as much enthusiasm as a sloth.

"We all get to build a part of the whale, and the teacher is going to put it on the ceiling above the hall. It's going to be really neat," EmmaGrace said with an almost dreamy tone, imagining a 50-foot humpback whale floating above her as she walked to her classroom every day.

Her one wish in life was to become a mermaid, and I had no doubt that her imagination had sent her under the waves swimming alongside that whale. As EmmaGrace reported the happenings of her school day, I responded with "Really" and "Wow" until we were back in the garage. I was entirely grateful that EmmaGrace hadn't notice my lack of conversation masked by strategically placed one-word comments to keep her going. Before opening the car door, I mustered the strength to stand up straight and walk by her side into the house. She hung up her backpack on the hook inside the door and plopped down for a snack. Ron whooshed in behind the counter, and I headed for the familiar comfort of the pea green couch where there was nothing to do but rest. The phone rang and based on how Ron slipped into the pantry and shut the door, I surmised that he was talking about me. It was Suzannah calling to try and help Ron process what was happening. When he was done, he handed the phone over to me.

"Hi," I weakly whispered.

"How are you doing?" she asked already knowing the answer.

I rattled off a list of laments followed by Suzannah reminding me over and over, "If you feel that bad, imagine how the cancer feels."

She knew it was little comfort but didn't have much else to offer her sister who was unlikely to beat the odds.

After I hung up, I noticed a distinct shift in Ron's demeanor. He was a Type AAA+++ personality, normally very high-strung and unable to stop overachieving in everything he did. During our marriage I had gotten used to being low man on the totem pole of his activity list and found deep enjoyment in hanging out with my kids, watching them discover new things each and every day as they walked on the planet for the first time. I found it incredible that so much of what we took for granted was novel to them and was awestruck by their daily amazement. They were clearly teaching me mindfulness in a way no therapist could. Ron, on the other hand, couldn't sit still. His coping mechanism was never to stop moving. So, unless the girls were a part of building a bonfire or trailing behind him from one activity to the next, he was just a blur in and around the house. However, Suzannah must have pressed a button we didn't know he had because during that first weekend after chemo, Ron was relaxed, present, loving, funny, playful and considerate. The impact of his shift on my overall attitude was obvious to everyone. I settled in to be taken care of that weekend and felt truly happy for the first time since the war had been waged.

Sunday, November 20, 2005
On Sunday, my brother Phil hosted a brunch for family and friends. While I wanted to decline the invite, I just couldn't. It wouldn't be fair for the girls to miss out on fun and games with their older cousins. So, I put my own needs

aside and mentally prepared for the excruciating 50-minute drive to Mukwonago. Before leaving I debated with myself about whether or not to bring a bucket for the ride and decided against it, which then left me afraid that we'd have to pull over on that narrow, wooded road riddled with hairpin turns through the Southern Kettle Moraine Forest just so I could leave my breakfast on the shoulder. I opened the car door, sighed and plopped down on the front seat resigned to my fate. As we moved along the winding roads, I almost passed out. I normally would have enjoyed the beauty of the scenery, but on that day, agony prevailed. I groaned quietly to myself as my body protested, threatening to expel the acid sloshing in my stomach. Luckily, my will proved stronger, and we made it to my brother's without incident.

When we walked through the door, I was ready for bed. I forced a smile and squinted to focus on each well-wisher as I moved towards the bedrooms. I truly appreciated them but wasn't able to handle the interactions. Everyone moved in too close, and the hugs were almost painful. A long-time family friend who had recently finished his battle with prostate cancer wanted to impart his wisdom about how to handle what was to come. I focused intensely on his words, trying to pluck out something helpful from his experience. He reported that he had radiation seeds implanted to kill his prostate tumor. That was it. End of story. The room began to spin, and I imagined being in one of those after school movies of the1970's that tried to depict the disorienting feeling of taking drugs or alcohol. The voices talking to me were slowed, muddled to drawn out, incomprehensible sounds. Faces were blurry and oversized. The room felt like a merry-go-round I had to escape before I threw up. I ducked into my brother's bedroom and collapsed on top of the guests' winter coats covering his bed. I closed my eyes trying to get my bearings and fell asleep.

Almost three hours later, I woke up feeling much better and wrestled myself free from the tangle of coats. Standing at the door, I took a deep breath and quietly crept back into the living room trying to go unnoticed. To my happy surprise, the party was beginning to disperse. Relief washed over me and quickly evaporated making way for the realization that I had to get back in the car if I wanted to go home. It was one of those necessary evils. Car sickness had always plagued me, and thanks to the chemotherapy, being a passenger became magnified to previously unimaginable degrees of cruelty. Luckily, I made it home without incident and dropped down on that all too familiar antique, pea green couch in the living room, letting my body melt into its cotton-filled cushions.

While I lay there, I realized I hadn't called any friends to let them know of my diagnosis. I felt as if I needed to but wasn't sure if I could. I volleyed back and forth in my mind whether or not I was ready to handle their responses before I decided to give it a try. I made a short list and sat at the kitchen counter where I could prop my head up during each call. I had a prepared dialogue to deliver and expected everyone to respond in much the same way but neglected to send them the script. There was no way for me to predict how difficult those conversations would prove to be. The word cancer caused some of my friends to say things so out of their normal lane, that they caught me entirely off guard. During that time, friends were the single most disappointing and rewarding part of my clash with cancer. New friendships took shape while old friends either dug their heels in to help or quietly slipped away. I called Jeff. He was one friend I hadn't spoken to in quite some time, but somehow I needed to connect with him first. He was a lovely soul, and when I heard his voice, I felt a leap of joy in my heart. He had nothing but words of encouragement for me.

"Remember, Joe. He had cancer at 26 and beat it. I expect nothing less from you. You're going to beat it," he said.

My next call was Cameron, another dear friend, who handled the news perfectly.

He said, "I can't believe it. How could someone so strong get cancer? Well, all I can say is I feel sorry for that cancer. It doesn't know whom it just took on. You're going to wipe the floor clean with it."

I loved that man and let out a chuckle because that was all I had the energy for, but inside I was laughing hysterically.

When I called my friends Mary and Debbie, they didn't have much to say but took immediate action regularly bringing food to the house. Mary was stealthy with her meals, quietly opening the front door, tiptoeing in, and leaving dinner on the counter without me even knowing she was there. On the other hand, Deb always stayed to chat, forcing me to eat in front of her. God bless her for making sure something nourishing was feeding my ailing body. On another call, I had to leave a message. My longtime friend Larry Mullen Jr. was on tour with his band, U2. I felt so awkward leaving him such a heavy message on voicemail, but I didn't know what else to do. I worried for a couple of days before he returned my call with a raw and honest reaction.

"I did get your message but just couldn't call back right away. I felt so much despair and didn't want to call feeling like that," Larry said.

We chatted briefly, and then I handed the phone over to Ron so Larry could feel more comfortable asking the questions he didn't want to ask me. After a few more calls from friends offering support, I was drained of every ounce of energy I possessed and once again collapsed onto the couch, which had become an essential part of my regular routine.

A couple days later, Larry surprised me when he called again to tell me that before the band was about to go onstage that weekend, one of his mates brought up his daughter who had been diagnosed with leukemia six months before my diagnosis. Along with her treatments, the doctors added a diet of specific foods known to stop the growth of blood vessels nourishing the tumor. Without new vessels the cancer cells would die. Stopping the growth of blood vessels was called anti-angiogenesis, and using anti-angiogenic foods, the eight-year-old girl entered remission earlier than the other kids diagnosed at the same time she was. In all honesty, I almost didn't absorb anything he was telling me.

"Can I find out more and get back to you later in the week?" Larry asked.

What else could I say but, "Of course."

After the call, Ron sifted through the untended pile of mail that grew daily. In it was an envelope addressed to me from Susan, a very old friend. Earlier in the week, I had run into her with her husband at the YMCA and blurted out my news. I didn't have the energy to choose my words carefully, so there was no real conversation. We just hugged, and I registered the look of shock on their faces. Over the years, Susan and I had often met for breakfast. She usually spent that time unloading her erratic emotions around a drug-addicted brother who kept showing up in the hospital emergency room where she worked as a nurse, her alcoholic mother who dished out regular unrest, and her marriage that wasn't what she hoped it to be. I listened over egg-white omelets and orange juice, helping her process her frustration. We had a comfortable, long-standing and very open relationship. So, when Ron handed me her letter, I wondered why she hadn't just called or stopped by.

Her note started with, "What devastating news! Steve and I remarked on how sad we felt at seeing you. Breast CA…. I'm not sure too many other words in the English language conjure up so much fear. You seem OK with it all…"

OK, note to everyone out there who knows someone diagnosed with cancer: Do not use words even remotely close to this. I understood it was hard to know what to say to someone who had been diagnosed, but she couldn't even spell the word out. I already knew it was devastating news…FOR ME. I wondered if she could imagine how it felt when *I* found out. Seriously?! That's right up there with another one people say, "God only gives you what you can handle." Is that right? Well then, God needs to replace his Kathy Bero calculator because the one He's using is seriously broken!

I did receive a follow-up note from Susan a year or so later. It was a little better but closed with, "Please know I'm with you in spirit and looking forward to seeing you someday all better."

Never did she call me or stop by to see me. Just those two oddly worded notes. When I ran into her some years later at a farmer's market, Susan gave me a heartfelt apology for her lack of friendship. She explained that she just hadn't been able to deal with everything going on in her life, and by that Susan meant having two healthy daughters. Geesh.

Other friends were lovely, and I appreciated their concern, but it was overwhelming to receive so many different emotions. Some tried to help by sending supplements, books, calling with alternative treatment ideas or referring me to new websites. Sometimes, they shared horror stories from other people they knew in my "situation" not realizing that every single cancer was different, not to mention that every body was different. I knew they were trying to provide some sort of motivational boost and loved them for it, but managing chemotherapy was about all I could handle. Family members also seemed to be at a loss for comforting words even though they tried very hard. One of my brothers-in-law called to provide his encouragement.

He said, "I hope you feel better soon."

Wednesday, November 23, 2005
Dr. Harper still hadn't received my results from one of the hormone receptor tests sent to Mayo Clinic. Without it, we were all growing a little tense. The test was very important in directing my treatment as it related to how the cancer used special proteins called hormone receptors. When progesterone and estrogen hormones attached to those receptors, the cancer grew. So, if the receptor status was positive, the cancer was treated in one way. If their status was negative, a different set of treatments was used. Typically, a woman with positive hormone receptors in her cancer had a slightly lower chance that cancer would recur after remission. Knowing the HER2/neu status was another way to identify a more effective treatment plan because cancer cells could also grab that protein to help them grow and survive. If the HER2/neu status was positive, there were chemotherapies designed to target that receptor, but the cancers tended to be more aggressive. Today, researchers are working on developing ways to design chemotherapy to look like those same proteins. In those studies, the chemo mimicked the hormone proteins, attaching to the cancer cells before being sucked in. The cancer "thought" it was there to help it grow, but really the protein was there to destroy it from the inside out. In that

way, the chemotherapy was also much less toxic to the body. As I learned more about the science, I added scientists to my list of prayers.

"Lord, give cancer researchers the information they need to save us without breaking our bodies or our banks."

Once my results from the ER/PR test had finally arrived, we were thrilled to know that it was positive for both. Unfortunately, the HER2/neu study looking at both the protein receptors and the number of genes in the cancer cells was botched and had to be re-run. The suspense of my hormone receptor status was killing not only me but my oncologist as well because a negative result meant fewer chemo treatments and possibly a different chemo all together. Nearly a week later, the lab at Mayo Clinic informed Dr. Harper that the second test had been botched as well. He was furious and couldn't hide it behind his calm demeanor. He was about to administer my second toxic treatment without knowing exactly what I was up against. Adding insult to injury, the lab had used up so much of my sample that they no longer had enough to conduct a third state-of-the-art HER2/neu study. So, after a few choice words from my oncologist, they fast tracked the third attempt and ended up with an ambiguous result, leaving Dr. Harper with no option but to employ the art of practicing medicine and make his own call one way or the other. He called it negative, which meant fewer doses of chemotherapy, and we both held our breath.

The second week of treatment was piled high with scans while I developed an aching pain in my neck and throat. Assessing my situation, the nurses concluded that there was no visible reason for my discomfort. However, I had a nagging voice in my head poking me to push them further. I squashed it down and got ready for another day of tests. Hannah took a ride to the hospital with me, so my parents could pick her up and take her somewhere more cheery.

As they started to walk away, Hannah cried, "Mommy coming? Mommy coming!"

I felt terrible. It was unnatural for her to be away from me so much.

I replied with a soft smile, "I'll be there in a minute."

Hannah didn't want to leave me but loved grocery shopping. So, my parents took my easily redirected two-year-old to wander through the aisles at Pick-n-Save. She never wanted to "buy" anything she just wanted to admire all of the colors lined up on the shelves. They would come back for me between the CT scan and the bone scan, which gave me a chance to get lunch while the injected radioactive tracers had a chance to settle throughout my skeleton. During the bone scan, the tracers would light up where I had cancer, giving my team of doctors a clear picture of any disease in my bones.

As I sat alone waiting for the technician, emptiness welled up again and filled my entire being. I wanted to take Hannah to the grocery store. I didn't want to shuffle down the institutional halls of the hospital to be swallowed up whole by another darkened room filled with pulsating monitors and humming machines. I forced myself to try my new practice of praying whenever I felt the oppression of cancer treatment squeezing me tighter. I prayed to be strong enough to stay the course for my daughters. If I made it, I would have lots of time to wander through the aisles with Hannah "oohhing" and "aahhing" over the mutli-colored boxes and cans of processed foods looking like stationary fireworks on the grocery store shelves.

When the technician arrived, she was clutching a metal box latched shut. She smiled weakly as if burdened by the heavy responsibility of injecting nuclear medicine into another human being, and I sat quietly until the needle, partially inserted into my bicep, hit something that blasted me with incredible pain.

"OUCH! WHAT JUST HAPPENED?" I yelled straining to keep my voice down.

"Oh, I must've bumped the needle up against a valve in your vein. It will likely be all right. I'll let the CT technician know in case there is a problem," she said dismissively but with a hint of cringe.

The sting caused tears to well up uncontrollably in my eyes as she pulled the needle out, leaving the catheter in. Without looking at me, she led me to the CT room where "Groovy Guy" greeted me. I dubbed him that because his appearance and demeanor threw me completely off-guard. His style was far from the polished, put-together look of the hospital professionals I had previously come in contact with. His hair was long and pulled back in a ponytail with a tiny little bun on the back of his head. A large hoop earring wiggled from his ear, and his sway-like swagger caused me to back away as he approached. Then, he called me "Sweetie."

"Hello, Sweetie. So we might be up against a valve I hear? Well, we'll give it a go, Sweetie. If blood doesn't come squirting out, we'll be all right, Sweetie."

It was all I could do not to lash out at him and keep from back handing that sweet, sappy smile right off his face. My pain was real and lasted throughout the entire scan, but no blood came squirting out, so apparently, that meant I was all right. As the day progressed, my entire body hurt. There was so much being done to me during those first two weeks that all of my pain receptors seemed to fire at the same time. It was pure chaos in my body, causing me to slip into weakness. I couldn't help but imagine the cancer growing stronger as I grew weaker. At lunch with my parents and Hannah, I could only watch them eat. My appetite had been wiped clean by the imagined difficulty of the impending bone scan. My parents pretended not to notice, and we all focused our attention on my happy little Hannah. Afterwards, they took me back to the hospital, and I asked them to wait with me in case my results were bad. It wasn't long before the radiologist appeared to enthusiastically report that the cancer didn't appear to have spread. Helpless to hold back the tears, my parents and I cried. It was the first piece of good news I had gotten since my nightmare began.

Happily, I breezed right through the bone scan. In the comparatively small room, I lay down on the table encircled by a metal donut-shaped machine. On my back, I studied a poster image of a serene tropical setting affixed to the ceiling above the scanning bed. Apparently, I was to imagine myself lying on the beach, tanning and sipping margaritas by the sea while the machine moved around me. When the scan ended, I shot off the table and sat in the hard plastic chair against the wall to wait for the radiologist who kindly hadn't made me wait long.

Dr. Yensing said, "While your skeleton lights up like a Christmas tree, I believe it's arthritis and not cancer. Now, I hope you'll be able to enjoy the rest of your day."

He brought the images up on the screen for me to see, and I was amazed by all the areas that were glowing. I thought arthritis was only in my knees, but clearly the disease was rampant throughout my body, working its way into my hips, neck and spine. Pre-cancer that diagnosis might have given me cause for concern, but on that day, it was just another thing not to worry about. I also reflected on how grateful I was that my medical team never made me wait for results, which went a long way towards quelling my continuous anxiety. With scans completed, my parents gave me a hug and took their leave. Hannah and I meandered through the maze of hospital halls back to the cancer center where we met Ron and EmmaGrace. I had organized for EmmaGrace to meet with the cancer counselor in hopes of getting some informed advice on how to work through my situation with her. When Claudia arrived, she introduced herself with a big smile and asked my eldest daughter if they could chat as she led her to a small room and closed the door. I slyly hung around eavesdropping through the paper-thin wooden door, listening to how quickly my daughter had assessed the situation and jumped into her expected role. Scenes from *The Hope Tree* took shape in her words. Clearly, the therapist had never read the book, or she would've recognized the dialogue immediately.

"I will be embarrassed when my mom's hair falls out."

"What will be embarrassing about that? Are you afraid people will laugh?" Claudia asked.

"No. There's also a lot of crying at our house," EmmaGrace continued as if verbalizing a list.

At the end of the session, she was asked to draw pictures of her family. Each one was happy and loving without a trace of sadness. When Claudia brought EmmaGrace out, Ron drove the girls home and I entered her office for a briefing by the confused therapist.

"EmmaGrace is very comfortable with expressing her feelings. You've done such a good job of being open and honest with what's happening. The kids in families like yours tend to do better over the long run," she said with an air of praise.

I laughed and said, "EmmaGrace is very good at reading a situation and picking up on what is expected of her. The statements she was providing you were direct quotes from a book we had read to her."

Claudia scrunched up her face, paused and said, "Well, just keep doing what you're doing and don't be embarrassed to talk about it."

I wouldn't have known how else to do what I was already doing. That's why I was already doing it. It would've been impossible to hide and whisper every time I had to talk about my day. Discussions about cancer and what I was doing to annihilate it were just part of our daily routine. It was one more of life's challenges that I intended to overcome, a blip on my screen of life. I wanted my family to feel comfortable talking to me about it because, let's face it, I was obviously different. There was no way to hide it. Why should I be embarrassed? Did I do something wrong that made me get cancer? It's not as if I asked for it. There was a school of thought out there that liked to pin it on the victim. I didn't subscribe.

I was very sore at the end of that day but relieved to get home into my own space where no one would stick me with a needle or strap me to a hard, 18-inch-wide table and slide me into the tubular mouth of one scanning beast or another. Unfortunately, by the time I got home, a barrage of emotional turmoil was overrunning our home, and on that night, my happy little girl cracked. As I tucked EmmaGrace into bed, she started to cry uncontrollably. I tried to hold her, snuggle as we always had and comfort her, but she wriggled away. I wished I had taken Claudia's number. I could've called her to ask her to tell me again just how well-adjusted my daughter was now that a microscopic cell called cancer had taken away even the most intimate moments between mother and daughter. Cancer was clearly going to leave no one in our family unscathed during its assault, least of all my children.

I was reminded that night that EmmaGrace had an intense ability to smell even the slightest scents. She could smell your breath and tell you what you had for lunch, so she most certainly would be able to smell the poison permeating my tissue. I smelled and tasted it every day. It was as if I was chewing on aluminum foil and drinking rubbing alcohol. I was repelled by it myself, but what was I to do? For me, there was no escape, but EmmaGrace could recoil from me, and she did. The growing gap between us brought such a profound sadness to my heart that after about 10 minutes of unsuccessfully calming her down, I gave up. I called for Ron, accepting that if I wasn't there, she might relax. When Ron entered the room, she immediately stopped crying as I dragged myself out, feeling dejected and useless, but careful not to show it. I wanted my girls to see me as brave and strong, a model for tackling life's challenges both big and small. Glancing back over my shoulder as I crossed the bedroom door threshold, I saw my vulnerable little seven-year-old girl downcast and picking at her sea-foam green sheets. She was drowning in her own sorrow and grief, never mind my own.

Thursday, November 24, 2005
The next day was Thanksgiving, and I woke up feeling pretty great. It had been nine days since my first treatment, and the effects were waning. The smell of cooking sausages wafted up to my bedroom, drawing me out and down to the kitchen where Ron was making egg muffins for breakfast. It smelled heavenly, but my sense of taste betrayed my sense of smell. With that first bite, a wave of nausea passed through me as my mouth watered uncontrollably. I took the muffin and scraped the scrambled egg off and tossed the rest away. I found it impossible to find food that tasted appealing to my taste buds, which were fried by the toxic assault, but scrambled eggs were non-offensive. I could eat them without any real physical reaction, and they gave me the boost of energy I needed to prepare in anticipation of my family arriving later that day to feast.

After breakfast, Ron gave Hannah a bath while EmmaGrace and I picked up toys and mopped the floors. After Hannah's bath, Ron turned to cutting wood for the bonfire and prepared the turkey. By the time my parents arrived, Hannah was down for a nap, and I would've hollered "Score!" if I had had any energy left. My mom and dad burst through the front door laden with festive energy and loaded down with pans of stuffing and sweet potatoes. They rolled up their sleeves and dove into helping make creamed spinach and pecan pie. I tried not to be useless but failed miserably. My sister-in-law Jo brought mashed potatoes, apple and pumpkin pies, and her much-loved chocolate chip cookies. Throughout the night, I sat slumped against my dad on the couch forgetting to worry about whether or not Hannah was eating actual food until she sauntered up to me in the living room, swaying with a little "aren't I adorable" head dip. She had an Andes Candy in each fist and one smeared across her face.

I asked, "Are you only going to eat sugar during the holidays?"

Hannah looked at her brown chocolatey, fist and gave a euphorically long-drawn-out, "Yesssss" through her sweet, candy-coated grin.

Firday, November 25, 2005
Black Friday brought new meaning for me that year. It was the day my friends Anne and Chris planned to take me wig shopping at Sharon's Wigs in Brookfield. My hair wasn't falling out in huge matted clumps yet, but it was falling out at a pretty good clip. Although I winced just below the surface, I kept a smile plastered on my face as we laughed with each style we tried on. There was the oversized 1950s blonde bouffant Dolly Parton wig, and the high-fashion dark bobs and wigs closer to my own naturally curly hair style.

The woman running the shop made a very gentle point to me as if to provide counsel.

"Can I make a suggestion?" she asked.

"Sure," I responded flatly.

"Usually women in your situation like to pick a wig that is very different from their normal hair, since it will be obvious to everyone it's not your hair no matter how good it looks," she asserted rather forcefully.

I stared at her and then at the wigs lining the shelves.

"I think it's best to just throw caution to the wind," she said smiling as she touched my arm.

I agreed and decided to think of the wig as a temporary makeover. After all, once the treatment was done, it would be two or more years before my hair grew back to its normal length, growing only six inches each year. So, I chose the newest styled auburn wig. It was short, and nothing my hair would've ever looked like. Anne suggested we buy hats, which made me pause, wondering why a bald cancer patient was expected to wear a hat or some other sort of head covering. Maybe buying hats was just an expression of solidarity among friends, or maybe it was a way to cover the uncomfortable reality of my situation? Either way, I acquiesced and purchased a camel-colored pill box hat, knowing I would never wear it.

We left the shop and met my parents for lunch at a Greek restaurant down the road where they used to take us as kids. We all sat in a booth, ate, swapped stories and laughed, providing me with another temporary reprieve from my ugly reality until I noticed the pain in my parents' eyes. They could only think about the possibility of losing me and found little humor in the conversation, so they took an early leave. I'm sure they thought they were ruining the moment, but on the contrary, it was cancer that had ruined that moment and every other moment.

At home, Hannah napped after a day of adventures in the woods with bonfires and stories of fairies. Ron and EmmaGrace were engrossed in the Johnny Depp version of Willy Wonka, so I opened the refrigerator door searching for something easy to make for dinner and settled on pasta with garlic butter.

After dinner, EmmaGrace asked, "Can I fix your hair, Mommy?"

I prickled with anxious fear. If I let her brush it, there was every possibility huge clumps would come out with each stroke. However, the desire to stay connected to my daughter overpowered my fear, and I was ultimately amazed that the majority held on. She made me up to look like Barbara Eden from *I Dream Of Jeannie*, as I relished the moment. If only I had been able to wiggle my nose and make the cancer disappear.

Over the next couple of days, the snow accumulated on the deck. I watched from the window as my girls, smiling through their chilled, red cheeks, worked to shovel it around and build tiny snowmen. Afterwards, they drank hot cocoa by the cozy bonfire while tears swelled from my eyes. Noticing me at the window, Ron successfully lured me out by spreading a thickly haired deerskin on the bench next to the fire pit, making me a little nest of warmth. Chemo brought on many changes in my body, one of which was the inability to get warm. My normally hot body was cold all the time, but with the deerskin insulating my bottom and a warm fleece blanket wrapped around my top, the heat was sealed in fairly effectively. I put on a hat, knitted by my friend in Oregon, and pulled my hood over it, cinching it around my neck. On that night, I started the new activity of measuring my activity based on discomfort vs. benefit, and sharing that time with my family was worth the discomfort. There

56

was nothing better than watching my girls play together and watch out for each other. That simple thing meant more to me than it ever had before.

Bedtime came, and those contented thoughts melted away, leaving space for my anxiety to grow. The following day was treatment day. Just as I was finally starting to feel human again, chemo number two would snatch it away with another infusion of poison. I lay in bed planning how to organize my weeks around the side effects even though nothing useful came from it, because my days were what they were. Monday was chemo day; Tuesday was the Neulasta shot; and Wednesday, I would crash. Thursday through Sunday, I would be down and out, feeling as if death was a better option; and by the following Monday, I would pull myself out of the reaper's grasp and work hard to recover enough to be viable again. However, before I'd get there, I would have to start it all over again. That was my schedule. I hoped it would get easier with each treatment as Denise had said it would, but that was entirely laughable. I popped a Lorazepam and tried to sleep, but its effects were delayed. Instead of sleeping, my thoughts turned to our finances. Ron was a litigation consultant and hadn't had many billable hours since my diagnosis. Instead, he drove me to appointments and chased after kids, which worked out all right until I received my first invoice from the hospital leaving me stunned by the price tag of one month of treatment that may or may not save my life. I had already accrued more than $20,000 in bills and had a long road of treatment ahead of me. Luckily, before I got too far down the road of that line of thinking, the Lorazapam shut it down, and I fell asleep.

Monday, December 1, 2005
Unfortunately, in the morning, I woke up disheartened and right back where I had left off. I thought about how expensive my treatments were and couldn't see how we would be able to pay the bills. Each chemo treatment was somewhere around $10,000, and the second half would be even more. Then, there were doctors' fees, hospital fees, surgeries, radiation, medications, more appointments and tests.

Then, out of nowhere, I heard an otherworldly voice say, "Who cares about the bills. Beat the cancer and think about it then."

Thankfully, I was spared a true understanding of the total financial toll treatment would take on us because in just two years, my medical bills would total upwards of $500,000, which would've been a burden too heavy to carry in my vulnerable state.

In that moment, I began to understand the term "New Normal." It was a term that referred to life after a cancer diagnosis. Everything changed from your family life to your financial position to your outlook on death, and despite the heavy emphasis from my medical team to accept that change, I found it impossible to embrace. I was fighting for my "Old Normal" with every ounce of energy I could muster, and on that morning, I found a small bit of peace in what hadn't changed. EmmaGrace was up at 6:30 a.m. I took a shower, woke up Hannah and made breakfast for the girls. That much was still the same, but instead of racing out the door to take them to school, I quickly applied Emla Cream to the mediport area and taped Saran Wrap over the white, pasty dollop to keep it from rubbing off on my loose-fitting shirt. Emla Cream was my new secret weapon to combat the pain of the poke. It became a lifesaver each and every time the nurse inserted that oversized, curved needle through my skin and into the mediport to draw blood and deliver chemo. It truly provided a modicum of comfort in an otherwise difficult day. It was hard to deny the " New Normal," but I tried my best believing it was only temporary.

At the cancer center, they removed the Saran Wrap, cleaned the area, and then asked if I was ready. Since it was my first time using Emla Cream, I didn't entirely trust it. I looked the other way, took a deep breath and let it out slowly to reduce the pain from the impending poke. To my surprise, I only felt pressure as Lynn slowly inserted the needle. The beads of sweat forming on my forehead quickly evaporated, and I smiled. Once she had the vials filled, I was led through the friendly clinic halls lined with nurses flashing compassionate smiles my way. They made me want to be strong and worthy of their dedicated service, not wallowing in self-pity.

Judy, who loved dogs as much as I did, became my new chemo nurse, and that was our topic of choice. She met me at the door, walked through right behind me and went to work with a happy, chatty demeanor, asking the series of questions she would present at each and every visit.

"What is your pain level 0-10?"

"Where do you have pain?"

"Are you eating?"

"What and how much are you eating?"

"Are you sleeping?"

"Let's get you on the scale and see where you're at. OK?"

"Are you visiting with friends and family?"

"How are things at home?"

When she was satisfied that her list of questions was complete, Judy turned to the bag of saline hanging from the chrome hook on the wheeled pole and proceeded to flush the pic line through the mediport to clear out any blood clots that may have formed. While she performed her tasks by rote, she told me all about her dog. She asked about my dogs and then added the anti-nausea medication with Benedryl to my increasingly complicated cocktail. It was impossible for me to focus on her stories or what she was doing to me. I felt like that stupid girl in a horror film that just stands there screaming as her charming attacker chops her to pieces. It felt wrong to willingly take sedatives designed to make me docile while poisons were pumped through my veins, but I submitted anyway.

Dr. Harper arrived in the room before I was too far along in the poisoning. He examined my breast and lymph nodes for changes and almost leapt into the air. He seemed giddy as he reported that my skin was better and the tumor was changing. He was just thrilled that only one chemo treatment had caused palpable changes. It was a very good sign. When he left the room, I settled into the oversized reclining chair and imagined the cancer melting away like the Wicked Witch of the East in the *Wizard of Oz*.

Suzannah's words replayed in my head, "If you feel bad, think about what the cancer feels like."

I closed my eyes and thought about Ron and how he was becoming noticeably stressed and impatient with our situation. Once my treatment started, everything slowed down for him. Cancer was a waiting game, and I was receiving while everyone else waited. The doctors and nurses had it covered on the medical end, and my job was to take it lying down. Ron, on the other hand, had a whole different set of worries. Without the ability to get new work because he was needed at home, our bank balance was quickly dwindling, and he saw imminent collapse. We had to cover our daily living expenses along with the onslaught of prescription medications I ingested every day to keep me moving forward while at the same time paying our mortgage and feeding our babies. It had become very expensive to pay for my potential survival, and what if I died? Would it all have been worth it to him? I didn't dare ask him that question for fear he might say it wasn't. My fear of what I perceived his response to be caused me to withdraw from him and, for the most part, our conversations focused on the tasks at hand.

Tuesday, December 2, 2005

Neulasta day or "put-my-white-blood-cell-production-into-overdrive-day" had arrived. I dropped Hannah off with Ron's mom and went to K-Mart to pick up hats, gloves and toys for the school gift drive. I picked out a couple of Christmas presents for the girls and then drove to the cancer center to receive the ever-painful kick in the fanny Neulasta shot. Afterwards, I picked up Hannah, took her for a flu shot booster and cringed at the memory of my own poke. I had never really valued flu shots, but my precarious immune system required that we all got one. Afterwards, I refocused on Christmas shopping, which I viewed as my one critical responsibility next to living. Not wanting to drop the ball, I prepared myself for the task. My office was painted with burnt orange walls and white woodwork. It was a very cozy room, housing a collection of sculptures we had acquired in South Africa, but it was also one of the colder rooms in the house. To work at my desk in the winter, I had to dress in multiple layers. On that day, I started with a thermal long-sleeved top, then a flannel shirt and a zip-up polar fleece topped by a wool sweater. I just kept adding until I had the right combination of clothing and a comforting wave of warmth moved through my body like a good glass of whiskey. My muscles relaxed, and my shoulders dropped. I melted into the chair, absorbing the joy of giving as I clicked through a variety of toy websites.

By Wednesday, I could feel the Neulasta doing its work. My whole body ached as if I had a terribly high fever, and every joint throbbed with excruciating pain. I slumped at the dinner table, and as soon as everyone was done, I dragged myself to bed. The days following chemo number two were worse than before, forcing me to call Mary for another prescription. This time it was for Zofran, a very expensive anti-nausea medication. Ron picked it up on his way home, handed it to me and watched as I greedily swallowed it. Not long after, the nausea subsided but not enough to get me out of bed. For a full 24 hours, I lay there writhing in pain.

On Thursday, I had no reason to get out of bed. There was nothing for me to do but think, which led me to remembering the horses. I hadn't cleaned their stalls or given them hay for at least a few days, so I was grateful that the grass was still accessible in the pasture. The longer I lay in place, the greater my guilt became, leaving me no choice but to trick my debilitated body into feeling strong enough to drag itself downstairs. Without socks, I stepped into my winter boots, slipped my down parka over my jammies and headed for the barn. From the back door, the barn seemed so far away. I took a minute to imagine a gale force wind pushing me up the small hill towards the barn door and then pushed aside my deep desire to collapse in place and sleep before taking another step.

Out loud, I said to myself, "Keep moving forward."

In the barn, I was shocked to see the backs of both horses completely cloaked in icicles from a nasty storm the day before that I hadn't even been aware of. I scraped them down, picked the poop out of their stalls, threw some hay down from the mow and gave them each a scoop of grain. I rewarded myself by dissolving into their warmth, hugging their necks and asking them to give me strength. Simon and Boo, appreciative of the attention, sympathetically nudged me back with their noses. I longed to curl up in the corner of one of the stalls to nap before venturing out and back down the hill. Instead, I stumbled my way across the barnyard and into the house where I took a little rest before attempting to make stew for dinner. Pushing back at my compromised state, I gazed into the pot of chopped vegetables, boiling away on the stove when the phone rang. At that point in my treatment, I tensed with every call. It was very hard for me to participate in any kind of conversation, but my ability to focus while talking on the phone was nearly impossible. I remembered a radio interview I heard with Temple Grandin in which she talked about how hard it was for her to concentrate while looking at the person she was talking to. She focused much better on the phone as long as it wasn't noisy around her. It seemed I now had a better understanding of how she felt, but I was the opposite.

Reluctantly, I answered the phone and was pleasantly surprised by the caller. Julie, a parent at EmmaGrace's school, had organized a dinner tree for us and explained when meals would be at school for pickup. I was overwhelmed with affection for her and wanted to tell her I loved her. I hardly knew her, but my emotions were at such a heightened state and, thanks to chemo, my filter was lost and would, unfortunately, not return until 2015. Blurting out my feelings of the moment was often uncontrollable and terribly awkward for all involved, so luckily, I had the strength to resist at that moment and hung up the phone. As soon as I did, it rang again. It was Deb calling to check in. Her husband, Jim, was the pastor at one of the three Lutheran churches in town, but he didn't really fit in. He was brilliantly witty, and most of his sermons soared over the heads of his parishioners. Deb was calling on Jim's behalf.

"Jim asked me to call and see when a good time would be for him to come over and pray with you?" she said without even asking if I wanted to pray with Jim.

The reaction I had was viscerally repulsive. I couldn't understand why he wanted to do that. I could still get out to church if I wanted to. Without answering and leaving her hanging, I continued my thought process. Was he thinking he'd give me my last rites? Wasn't it a little premature for that? Of course, that wasn't at all what he had in mind, but I couldn't get past the possibility.

"I'm fine, Deb. I don't need him to come over, but thanks for asking," I answered trying to sound gracious.

I hung up feeling defeated, scratched an itch on my head, and as I pulled my fingers away, a clump of hair came with them. Then, later that day, in an act I can only describe as defiance, EmmaGrace walked up to me and tugged on my hair.

I snapped, "MY SPACE!"

Her eyes watered, and she ran to Hannah. I felt terrible. I was mostly trying to protect her from nightmares with clumps of my hair in her little fists, but it also hurt. My scalp had become extremely sensitive, even painful. All of my senses were heightened in a painfully strange, chemically induced sort of way.

I worked to push the ache back by looking for peace out of my living room window, studying the many acres of prairie I had restored some six years before and reflecting on happier times.

The receding glaciers of so long ago had sculpted an awe-inspiring landscape riddled with hidden streams, meandering between two drumlins, and I got to live there. The vibrant prairie graced their gentle slopes, washing them in purple, orange, yellow, red, white and blue during the warm months when the flowers were in full bloom. Drought years never seemed to affect the plants that drew up water from the springs running continuously just beneath the surface. My perspective and appreciation of nature's intricate beauty had heightened as well. Some mornings, I sat alone in the house staring out the window and getting lost in the pink and orange sky as it grew with the sunrise. The silhouette of a silo adjacent to four large trees sitting atop the neighboring drumlin dominated the scene. It was as if I was taking in my own private art show. The snow-covered ground twinkled as it enhanced the natural relief of the landscape. I considered the shrubs, trees and animal dens, along with the bonfire pit and toys left in the yard, marveling at how they all looked like a ghostly copy of themselves under the blanket of snow. It was a painting that missed nothing. I took in the beauty one more second and then sighed. It was time for a shower, which meant more hair in the drain. I hadn't taken a shower the previous day just so I could keep a little more hair just a little bit longer even though the little bit that was left was terribly matted against my head, making me look like a dog with mange. Adding to the mess, I wore a hat to bed, so the loose hair wouldn't end up in piles on my pillow because, most likely, it wasn't even attached to my scalp anymore.

I stood up from my chair and emphatically announced, "I love my family and my life. No cancer is going to take that away! Keep moving forward."

Being mugged was a concept that came to me often. While I had been blessed to have never experienced it first hand, succumbing to the violation of prescription drugs, groping medical hands, unwanted needles and cancer gave me a connection to all those strong women who had beaten the crap out of their muggers. When I was in South Africa, I was told a story about a group of nuns who had learned the martial arts. One nun was attacked. I don't remember her circumstances, but she left her attacker crumpled on the ground. That's who I wanted to be with this cancer, egging it on until it lost its will.

"Is that all you've got? Well, I've got more!"

The words were always the same, whether I was weak or strong, and became one of several mantras I used to push myself forward.

As I mentioned earlier, the term "brave" was a familiar label for people in cancer treatment. At the start of my treatment, I hated all of those labels, but something clicked for me after the second treatment. People really do have to be brave to walk into the cancer clinic and willingly accept a dose of poison that had killed others before them. Every day had become an act of bravery for me. Was I going to get out of bed? Was I going to take the medication prescribed? Was I going to submit to more tests? Was I going to open my veins to another round of my customized toxic cocktail? Everything I did was an intentional action. I did nothing thoughtlessly, trying to preserve my valuable energy stores and careful not to waste them on something pointless. Each and every day became a series of strategic decisions made with my compromised mental capacity. I was practicing mindfulness, without even knowing it.

Saturday, December 6, 2005
And so, the time had come. Too much hair had fallen out. We dropped the girls off at school, and Ron took me to the wig shop to collect my order. It was a surreal experience. By making me look completely different, that wig would provide me a weird sort of anonymity I was not prepared for. I would soon discover that I could walk into a store where the clerks knew me by name before my diagnosis but wouldn't recognize me at all as a cancer patient. In some venues, the loss of my hair would make me invisible, which brought both a sigh of relief on the days I wanted to complete my task without interruption and utter loneliness even still.

With the wig in the bag, Ron drove me to my parents' house. He put a chair in front of the bathroom mirror, and I stood staring at myself for several minutes before I heaved a breath in and then out as I plopped down on the chair.

"Are you ready?" Ron asked a bit sheepishly.

"I don't have a choice," I replied feeling crushed.

I had already lost my normal life, and it was time to say good-bye to my normal hair as well. As the razor traversed my sensitive scalp, I cried. I cried from the pain. I cried from the loss. I cried from the injustice.

Ron struggled. He kept asking if he should stop. If he had, I would've had one bald side to my head and one zombie-like. In a better state of mind, I might have laughed, but I wasn't there. I just wanted it over and begged him to keep going. I watched in the mirror as dull matted hair cascaded down my face and fell over my slumped shoulders. When just the stubble remained, I asked Ron to leave me alone. I stood there taking in my face, which had also changed. The meds had made it puffy. As the woman at the wig shop had promised, I was definitely getting a makeover, but it was not the look I would have chosen and certainly would've paid handsomely to avoid. I wanted to look normal again, but the only way to go back was to keep moving forward. My intellectual thoughts pushed my emotions to the back seat, and I plopped the wig on, twisted it slightly into place and opened the door. At that time, I didn't know I could've had it cut to fit my face, which might have made it look a little more natural. Instead, I took it for what it was and wore it without ever even combing it. What a sight I must've been. I opened the door and walked into the kitchen where my parents were waiting.

"Oh, it looks nice, Honey," my mom said maintaining a loving smile.

"It really does," my dad added.

Neither one of them was convincing, but I appreciated their attempt. Then, my mom asked if they could see my head. Her request came totally from left field.

"Really?" I asked, thinking I didn't want to take the energy to reposition the wig again.

They both nodded yes. My mom looked nervous and supportive. My dad was just anxious. I removed the wig and stood there. Then, I turned away and went back to the mirror to quickly reposition my hair hat. I came to hate that wig. It itched and made my scalp sweat along with causing me to flush, which I later learned had nothing to do with that wretched wig. I was just suffering from one more side effect, having been thrown into immediate menopause by the toxic chemo soup.

Noticeably upset, my mom followed me to the bathroom and began to cry.

"I was supposed to get this. Not you. You have small children," she sobbed.

"But I'm stronger and younger than you. I'll beat this. It would've been harder for you, and I need you," I sincerely said trying to comfort her as I felt the adrenaline move through my body and boost my strength.

"But I've lived my life," she continued as if there was a choice.

"No, you still have another 30+ years to go and great grandchildren to meet. It's better that I got it. I'll beat it. I promise," I said with complete resolve.

"I know you will, Honey," my mom said as she enveloped me in her loving embrace.

I had no other way to comfort her than not to show my own pain. To do that honestly, I had to believe without a doubt that I would prevail and meet my own grandchildren someday. Society had us programmed to be solemn around cancer, but with the survival rates growing, I didn't want to be solemn. I needed to stay strong, positive and look for ways to kill it, preventing its recurrence not just treating it. I needed to take another step forward.

Mid-December 2005
I tried to stay connected to the "normal world," and in one week dragged myself out to coffee with friends, hosted Ron's aunt for a short visit and took care of Hannah in the afternoons. Oddly enough, in my new normal, that proved to be completely overdoing it. Visiting had become more exhausting and debilitating than almost anything else. Aside from trying to make conversation, it felt as though people thought they were seeing me for the last time – a reading of my last social rites – if you will. Without considering the mental toll it would take, I decided to cut off most social contact.

Before my third chemo treatment, Larry was working to connect me with a doctor in Boston, Massachusetts, who was very knowledgeable about anti-angiogenic compounds being used to make a specific chemotherapy. Larry asked him to talk with me about one called Avastin that wasn't approved in the United States for my cancer but was being used successfully in other parts of the world. After a short conversation on the phone, Dr. Li offered to send me a booklet, listing different foods and their special compounds. As I leafed through its pages of charts and scientific names, I couldn't help but notice how something that would have been easy for me to interpret before my diagnosis, had become a foreign language with unrecognizable characters. I stopped on one page that had a word I did recognize – cranberry. Since I struggled to process the information in the chart associated with the entry of cranberry, I settled on being satisfied with just knowing it was listed. The entry of cranberry in that booklet was enough to start me thinking that my recent cravings for the little red Wisconsin-grown fruit were my body telling me I actually NEEDED the fruit, and while it was Dr. Li's contention that I could help myself by eating foods that fought cancer, my body clearly already knew.

I called Suzannah to share what was for me very exciting, and although she was skeptical, she advised, "Try it all. You don't want to get to the end and say, I should've."

Riding on that wave of excitement, I asked a doctor friend of mine, who was a graduate of the Andrew Weil Integrative Medicine Program, to connect with her network to see if there was agreement on cancer-fighting foods. I was looking for corroboration from a trusted source. What she reported back to me was a big surprise. It was a resounding "stick to the treatment protocol." I tabled the booklet, deciding it was just too much for me to process while grappling with overwhelming fatigue. Sadly, I put the idea of using food to fight cancer away and hunkered down in place, taking care of Hannah as much as possible, which ultimately proved to be easier than I had anticipated. We had unwittingly set up our first floor perfectly to accommodate the co-existence of a sick mommy and a busy two-year-old. From the couch, I could watch Hannah at her project table, toy box or music station. While she happily played, I used that time on the couch to talk with research doctors about other ways I could help myself fight cancer, which meant I was on the phone a lot.

One day Hannah insisted, "No tone, Mommy!"

Feeling as if my wrists had been slapped, I vowed to only use the phone when she was asleep.

When I spoke with scientists and doctors about my case, I found that they provided so much technical information that it became nearly impossible for me to process it all. I hadn't yet realized that "chemo brain" had already set in. Writing and reading had become very difficult and mostly out of the question given that chemo was also affecting my eyesight. I struggled verbally, and my ability to put coherent sentences together was waning. It was as if I was too tired to finish a thought out loud, and my sentences were left to taper off and linger in the ether. Sometimes, my thoughts were discombobulated as they traveled beyond the boundaries of my vocal chords, but kindly, the brilliant people on the other end of the line didn't seem to notice. They repeated themselves or slowed their speech, clearly understanding my limitations. Out of respect for their time, I set a limit for myself on how long I would force them to endure my vocal malaise, and when my time was up, I graciously thanked them and hung up the phone. So, like attending a class, I took in their teachings over a period of time.

Ron picked EmmaGrace up from school most days, and by the fourth week of treatment, our days had developed a rhythm. Each one became a round robin of tasks, mostly with Ron and the girls moving around me. The dinner tree hosted by the parents in our new school was in full swing. Meals were left with EmmaGrace to bring home, and there was always more than we could eat. So, between the dinners and leftovers, we almost never had to cook. I was overwhelmed by the sheer kindness of people I had never even met, and I hungrily read their notes of encouragement. In the back of my notebook, I kept a list of what each person had sent, and a couple of times a week, I fired off thank you notes to push back at depression and remind myself that I wasn't alone.

My third chemo treatment of Adriamyacin and Cytoxan came and went. Despite my hypervigilance to stay away from germs, I contracted the stomach flu just in time for the Christmas season and my dad's annual excursion to see Santa with my girls. According to my dad, who "vetted" the santas at other malls, the one at Mayfair Mall in Wauwatosa was the most authentic. Christmas was his favorite time of year, and he loved the holiday wonder on a child's face. As far back as his time in the Army, my dad gravitated towards the profound joy he found in the sparkle of a child's eye. When stationed in England back in 1952, my dad made all the men in his platoon give up a portion of their pay to buy candy and toys for the kids in the orphanage. It was such an important event for my dad, that he mentioned it periodically throughout his life. So, who was I to put the kibosh on Santa?

With every ounce of energy in my reserves, I pushed back at the flu virus, smiled and agreed to go. My dad, it turned out, had gone above and beyond that year. The previous year, he had given EmmaGrace a bell on Christmas Eve and told her Santa had left it for her. Having seen the movie, *Polar Express*, EmmaGrace looked at that bell as a remarkable gift just for her and cherished it all year long. So, before our visit with Santa, my dad called the authentic looking jolly icon and asked him to remember her name. When we arrived at the mall, a line had already formed. We took our spot at the end, and with the wink of an eye, my dad subtly reminded Santa of their ruse, and then stepped back to sit on the adjacent bench and watch.

Several minutes later, we came around the corner of the Santa's workshop exhibit, and Kris Kringle exploded, "EmmaGrace! Do you still have my bell?"

Her face beamed with delight as she opened her hand to reveal the silver sleigh bell. Her smile was so bright that it blocked out the sun streaming through the sky lights overhead. She was clearly overwhelmed with the spirit of Christmas and couldn't believe Santa knew her name. She jumped into his lap shaking her bell and then gazed at his face with a goofy grin on hers. He just laughed and then turned his attention to Hannah. She was studying his lap but refused to sit on it. I glanced at my dad who shook like his own bowl full of jelly, laughing uncontrollably with Christmas cheer. My heart was warm as I looked at him and recognized that Hannah had to sit on Santa's lap to complete the experience, which meant I would have to sit on the corner of his chair. My shoulders dropped before I scooped up Hannah. I sat down, and her fingers went right into her mouth as she worried through the whole two minutes. Her sister, on the other hand, couldn't stop smiling. It was the best thing she had ever experienced. She chatted with Santa and recited her list of requests while my mom soaked up the merriment, standing nearby ready to step in if need be. Her affection for us was like a blanket of comfort always ready to swaddle us with her love and attention. She had such a grace about her that I wish I could've echoed with my kids.

With our time concluded and lots of other kids waiting in anxious anticipation, we said good-bye to Santa, collected our pictures and headed up to the play area next to the food court. My dad, still laughing to himself, took our lunch orders and headed to the deli counter. My mom shepherded Hannah around the slides while EmmaGrace bounced from one slide to another. I sat on the adjacent bench and closed my eyes for a brief minute, prying them open in response to the phrase, "Mom! Look at me!"

A woman sat down next to me, and I tried not to make eye contact with her. I knew I would have to chat if I did, and I was just too exhausted for that. I pretended not to see her as we sat in each other's personal bubble. My peripheral vision allowed me to note that she was staring at me the entire time. I had the wig on that day and knew I looked relatively normal, and yet, I felt terribly awkward. So, when I finally couldn't stand it anymore, I turned to look at her.

68

She sweetly smiled and said, "It looks good on you."

"What?" I questioned her, looking utterly confused.

"The wig," she continued. "My girlfriend has the same one."

For a moment, I didn't know what to say, and then I burst out laughing, "It must be the wig of the season. How is your friend doing?"

"She's hanging in there. I think she'll be all right," the woman said confidently. "How are you doing?"

"Holding my own, I guess. No one really knows yet, but I feel as if I am," I responded.

"Good for you. Keep believing. Gotta go," she said as she got up and walked away.

Laughing in disbelief at the oddity of our conversation, I tried to understand what had just occurred. She didn't have any kids playing there, and when I looked for her through the bustling crowd of shoppers, she was nowhere to be found, leaving me to question whether she had ever been there at all.

December 23, 2005
Because of my extreme discomfort, activity in general was accompanied by overwhelming distress. It was the holiday season, and there was no escaping my obligations. I was either at doctor's appointments or visiting with family. The non-stop action came to a head on the eve of Christmas Eve when I finally broke down. EmmaGrace's Christmas enthusiasm pushed me over the edge, and humiliated by my response to her love of the holiday, I called my parents in to rescue her. They always embraced the true spirit of Christmas and whisked my eldest away for an overnight, which was probably as much therapy for them as it was for her. I had anticipated that the following day, Christmas Eve, would be even harder for me and braced for the worst, but apparently, I had received an early gift. The new regimen I had put into play to beat back the side effects of cancer treatment seemed to be working. Starting two days before chemo, I took in eight ounces of Kefir twice daily. One day before chemo, I started taking Pepto Bismol three times a day, and acidophilus twice while drinking organic milk all day long. To that I added Nexium for acid reflux and two steroid pills for good measure. The witching hour by the previous three treatments should have been 8:30 a.m. on Christmas Eve, but nothing of note happened. I had the mandatory fatigue and slightly nauseous stomach, but all in

all it seemed the new plan was working. However, with the yin there's always a yang and fewer frantic trips to the bathroom led to my heightened irritability. I was so crabby without the distraction of frequent vomiting, that it was actually harder to stay positive. I snapped at every little thing and cried uncontrollably all day long. Merry fricken' Christmas to me. My body, mind and spirit were again breaking down. No matter how hard I tried to stay positive, bursts of anger came from out of the blue and overwhelmed my entire being.

I called my oncologist to complain, "What's wrong with me? I feel completely out of control."

Dr. Harper worked to quell my anguish, "I know it doesn't seem fair, but everything you're going through is part of the chemo ride. Pretty much everyone goes through it, but at varying degrees. You're no different, but it will end. It really will."

Helpless to change my situation and hard pressed to see how I was going to survive a ride like that, I took his words to heart. I didn't want to be like everyone else. I wanted to be different, but clearly what I wanted was not part of the cancer treatment equation.

Ron drove Hannah and me to my parents' house where we joined EmmaGrace to celebrate the birth of Jesus with the rest of my family. I walked in through the laundry room and directly into the family room where their brown leather couch sat empty just waiting for me to collapse into its deep, down-filled cushions. I closed my eyes before saying hello to anyone and felt almost euphoric as the familiar smells, joyful sounds and holiday spirit engulfed my broken spirit. Each year, my parents' cooked or baked for days to create one of their most cherished gifts, a huge spread of delicious small plates and delightful treats. It was also a strategic gift, distracting the kids with a constant stream of holiday fare while giving the adults time to chat before the presents under the tree were just too hard to resist. The menu for the night rarely changed, and every cell in my body was immediately transported to happier times. I set my mind to sampling everything, and Ron kept plates of food appearing at regular intervals on the coffee table in front of me. I refused to be cheated out of what could've been my last Christmas Eve with family, so I sampled shrimp, artichokes, stuffed mushrooms, cocktail sandwiches and more. Even though the flavors were distorted by my compromised taste buds, I nibbled anyway relying entirely on my tongue's muscle memory. I appreciated my family treating me as if nothing was different even though I drifted in and out of sleep to the comforting sounds of my nephews leading a game of hide-n-seek with the girls while my dad played Christmas carols on the piano. After the packages were opened, we expressed gratitude, sang carols, and told stories until it was time to

70

go home. In a normal year, I would've eaten my way through the evening and tumbled satiated into the car, where I would lean my head against the window to watch the night sky for any sign of Rudolf's red nose glowing amidst the stars. I had been doing that same routine my entire life and loved including the girls in my own personal little tradition. For them, I found a star or planet twinkling red in the night sky and announced that it was Rudolf on his way to our house.

"Look! There he is! We better get in bed fast when we get home," I would sing out.

They would flatten their little noses against the car windows searching the sky and exclaim, "There he is! I see him!"

On Christmas Eve, 2005, I leaned my head against the window and with closed eyes mustered the energy to declare that Rudolph was "right up there" on his way to our house. It was weak, but they didn't seem to notice in their anticipation of our routine. When we arrived home, the girls scurried off to bed with Ron on their heels. I pulled out the presents from their hiding place, and when he reappeared, we wrapped some and set up the others so they were ready for play in the morning. We filled the space under the tree with colorful boxes and oversized bows and then stuffed their stockings, which my mom had made over countless love-filled hours the year they each were born. When it was all done, we would normally have had a cocktail in front of the tree with Christmas music playing softly in the background, but Christmas Eve on chemo wasn't the same. I only managed to hang in there until the presents were under the tree, and then I left Ron alone, dragging myself upstairs and collapsing into bed.

December 25, 2005
Christmas morning came too soon. EmmaGrace was up at 7:30 a.m., but because it was too early to wake Hannah, we snuggled in bed and chatted about what Santa might have left for her. I felt the warmth of that moment deep in my soul and wanted time to stand still, but when the clock struck 8:00, EmmaGrace launched out of our bed and scurried off to drag her little sister from her crib. The excitement exploded. Hannah was already dialed in to the material benefits of the holiday, taking cues from her big sister. Their first stop was the stockings hanging on the banister outside of their rooms. Hannah studied her sister's actions for a moment and then poked her hand in, picking out one item after another. When EmmaGrace dumped hers on the ground, Hannah did the same, diving into the chocolate and peppermint treats that were hidden down deep in the toe. After a few minutes, the stockings lost their appeal, and the girls, with wide grins, pleaded to see what Santa had brought them. By that time, Ron had already gone down to make coffee and set up the camera. I built suspense by

71

asking what they thought Santa had left as I slowly made my way down the stairs, reminding them to stay at the top.

After several suspenseful seconds at the bottom while I confirmed that the camera was on, I looked into the living room where the tree stood and exclaimed, "Oh, my goodness! Look at what Santa left! I just can't believe it!"

"Can we come down? Please!" EmmaGrace screeched with a wild smile.

"Girls, come on down and Merry Christmas!" I exclaimed.

I stood at the bottom of the stairs unable to move, having already used up most of my energy stores at the stockings. My chest was heavy, and my breathing was labored as if I had just finished running a race. The girls almost trampled me as they flew down the stairs like homing pigeons programmed to recognize their own special present under the tree. Hannah was over the moon with her *Tommy The Train* set, and EmmaGrace squealed over her doctor kit. I sat in a chair opposite the tree and searched for joy in their sparkling eyes. We opened a few more presents before I collapsed once again onto that all too familiar pea green couch with eyes closed, only opening every minute or so as if to take a snap shot of the scene.

Once our morning was complete, we cleaned up and rebooted for the next celebration at Ron's folks. Christmas day was always wild with the cousins, nine in all, ages ranging from one to fifteen years old. I picked a chair as far out of the fray as possible while still being present and struggled to sit upright as I drifted in and out of sleep seemingly unnoticed. After the presents were opened, dinner was served, and the kids settled in to play with their loot. I would've joined the other adults on the quiet and cozy three-seasoned porch heated by a gas fireplace, but Suzannah and I went upstairs instead so she could examine my breast. She was so curious to see if the tumor could be felt, but it was nowhere to be found. We talked about the looming mastectomy surgery and where I was with my treatment, and even though she was describing the amputation of my right breast, her word choices always put my mind at ease.

"Dr. Doering has done thousands of mastectomies, so there's nothing to worry about there. He will cut out as much breast tissue as he can and also take the lymph nodes under your arm. The nodes will be sent to pathology while you're still on the table to assess which ones and how many, if any, contain cancer. That's really important information, which will tell them if you need to have more treatment. But the fact that your tumor is impossible to feel anymore, I think it's a good bet that the chemotherapy is working," she said encouraging me to stay positive.

I held her hopeful attitude while I was in her orbit, but on the drive home, I became overwhelmed by that familiar feeling of erupting anxiety. I popped a Lorazepam and settled back in my seat, not willing to be robbed of that one moment of peace that I had worked so hard to find.

December 26, 2005

Ron took the girls out to play, and I felt depression gain another foothold. All of my energy had been given over to the holiday festivities, and I had no strength left to stave off the ominous negativity. While my family played outside, I cried into the cream-colored, suede pillow accenting the pea green couch and drifted into sleep once again where I knew I would feel nothing. It had become my most reliable defense mechanism, leaving conscious emoting behind.

I was roused awake by my own voice asking out loud, "Would you feel better being outside with the kids or slipping in and out of sleep on this damn couch?"

The answer was obvious. Physically it seemed nearly impossible to get up, but I mustered the strength to put my winter clothes on and walk outside to the deck, making it as far as the lounge chair Ron had brought out of storage and planting myself as I heaved each breath. I watched the energetic happiness bounce all around the yard while Ron taught the girls how to navigate his Christmas gyro car over the snowdrifts. Once the allure wore off, the girls called for sledding, and Ron helped me into the cab of the truck and then tossed the red plastic sleds into the bed. He skillfully drove through the deep snow sliding all the way to the hill on the south side of our land where I reluctantly went down one time with each of them. It was an incredibly laborious process because Ron had to pull me back up the slippery hill in between rides. By my third time down, I had nothing left and sat in the truck with the heater blasting. Family sledding should've brought me great delight, but instead I felt nothing but sadness.

Around that time, I started to talk out loud to myself…a lot. I almost never talked with anyone else unless I had to. It just used up too much energy, and my thoughts felt necessarily private. I almost became like my own coach, for example, telling myself to accept any and all help with meals. There was nothing that unburdened me more than knowing all I had to do was take something out of the freezer and pop it in the oven. Voila! Dinner! I reminded myself I couldn't do it all – obviously – and had to put my energy into getting better. I reminded myself to take a shower, take my medication and make necessary phone calls. Every day, I forced myself to listen to meditation and mindfulness CDs, my favorite of which was a series by BelleRuth Naparstek. Her affirmations about how healthy I was seemed to put a productive spin on closing my eyes, making me feel as if I was doing something to move myself closer to normal. It was hard at times to embrace the affirmations which felt disingenuous, but I did it anyway.

Eventually, my attitude shifted away from pity for myself, and I planned to see an end to my horror by July 2006. I laid out benchmarks, projecting forward to help me stay focused on recovery week after week even though I was still taking chemotherapy. I presented a list of questions to my doctors at each appointment, which gave me critical points to focus on and plan around each month, and as much as they didn't love my list, they entertained me anyway. The side effects of the chemo drugs were mounting. Constipation, mouth sores, neuropathy in my fingers and toes, extreme fatigue, trouble breathing, distorted hearing and painful eyes were added to my daily challenges. Each side effect came with the introduction of more medication. It never seemed to end. I thought about those shows depicting cancer patients with a pharmacy at their bedsides. That's where I was. I trusted my doctors and embraced their philosophy of not thinking about how those drugs might be synergistically affecting my body. All I wanted was relief in any way I could get, it and if the doctors gave it to me, I believed it would work. Unfortunately, relief from the side effects of one medication brought on different side effects that required another medication to counteract those side effects, which then brought on more and so on. The vicious cycle was in full swing, and my vital organs were paying a heavy price. Once in a while, I felt a distant inkling that the harm created by all of that medication might be greater than the good, but our doctors pledged to "do no harm," so I ignored my inner voice and kept plowing ahead.

I hadn't yet implemented the new food "plan" Larry had brought to me because the booklet I was given was too researchy, and it was just too hard for me to process. I did, however, start to make my own list of foods based on more digestible information that I found on the Internet or had garnered from discussions with a food scientist from Louisiana State University in Baton Rouge. Dr. Jack Losso advised me to eat produce I almost never ate and definitely didn't know how to cook. He talked to me about cooking techniques that preserved disease-fighting compounds and gave me an opportunity to learn something new about using food as medicine. While I would've loved to have absorbed all of what he was teaching me, my energy stores were depleted, leaving me to table the anti-angiogenic food list and settle back into pharmaceuticals while trying to hold my own each and every day.

One day Ron stated, "It might be good if you cleaned a room here and there when you can until the house is done."

Holding my own became nearly impossible and was made even more so by Ron's own lack of normal. He didn't know how to handle our state of affairs and seemed to believe that I could do more to help around the house. Sadly, we rarely talked about our feelings or emotional needs, choosing to economize our energies and stick to what was necessary for getting through each day, but that only made our lives harder. My perceptions were skewed, leaving me incensed over the insanity of him thinking I could do even a little bit of work around the house.

Observing him through my own wretched shroud, I grumbled to myself about how his stress load was tiny compared to mine.

"How am I supposed to do that? I can barely sit up most days. My job is to fight cancer. Isn't that good enough?" I said, spitting venom his way.

Ron was visibly taken aback and explained, "No! That's not what I mean. You misunderstood me as usual. I just feel bad that you're lying around feeling sick and thought if you did a little bit of work when you could, you'd feel better. I always feel better when I'm useful."

Of course, I had entirely misunderstood what Ron was trying to do for me. He was actually feeling sorry that my condition had left me with the inability to help in any way and projected his own feelings onto me. In a typically male way, he hoped being busy would alleviate any guilt I felt over doing nothing. From my perspective, doing nothing was the only thing I could do well at that point. Clearly, he misjudged my mental state but not out of malice. Cancer treatment twisted the way I perceived situations and intentions, making my interactions with people almost surreal. I lost patience as I never had before and cried every single day. In hindsight, the problem was that the caregiver was often overlooked, and it was impossible for me to see Ron's perspective at that time. In truth, he was under more stress than I was. I was working to live; but if I died, that would be that. However, the possibility of my death brought on a whole host of new challenges for him as he tried to take care of the present and prepare for the future.

Outside of the house, I joked around and made light-hearted comments to help others feel comfortable with my weakening state, but at home it was a different story.

One day, EmmaGrace said to Ron, "I wish God hadn't given Mommy the cancer gene. She's so crabby."

I felt terrible and once again resolved to dragging myself out of the quagmire of self-pity and shoring up my attitude, which was a routine that had become as much a part of my day as eating. Even with the Naparstek exercises, I felt put upon by the world. I had to consciously work to keep the emotional pit of

75

cancer at bay, and one way I did that was to dive deeper into research on anti-angiogenic drugs. Suzannah had already made sure I was taking Celebrex, which was anti-inflammatory as well as anti-angiogenic, and the anti-angiogenic chemo Avastin was still hanging out there as a possibility for me. Dr. Harper was already using it on other cancers, but was not familiar with its use on inflammatory breast cancer. I asked him to check into a small study on Avastin, done by the National Institutes of Health (NIH) on inflammatory breast cancer. He contacted one of its researchers who explained that the study showed an extension of life by months for IBC patients, but it had not yet been approved. Unfortunately, Avastin, like so many other critical medications, was shelved for use on the cancer I hosted because of the arduous United States approval process that tests a drug on each and every type of cancer. Even drugs widely used in other countries had to go through the FDA approval process, which could take up to a full decade to complete. It was frustrating for doctors who were familiar with shelves of drugs that had successfully demonstrated their use in other countries, and yet they couldn't get their hands on them to help their own patients because of government limitations or legal disputes.

I decided I could break those shelves and spill life-saving medications into the hands of those who needed them, namely myself, and even though Avastin cost close to $15,000 per dose, I felt desperate to have it. I had no idea how I would pay for it, but I knew I needed it. Dr. Harper supported me, as he always did, and somehow got my insurance company to pay for the drug. I felt blessed to be one of approximately 10,000 people around the world who were using Avastin at that time and felt sure it was my ticket to freedom. From Dr. Harper's point of view, I had nothing to lose, so he added it to my second set of dose-dense chemotherapies, and I looked forward to the new year. Adding it to my toxic cocktail was sort of a jumping off point for me into self-advocacy, which meant thinking more critically and intentionally about my own treatment. Each time I questioned, I seemed to move one step closer to recovery.

New Year's Eve 2005
Conversations with me, myself and I continued with simple reminders like, "Cancer doesn't follow rules. You're doing everything right by leaving no stone left unturned. You don't typically go easy on yourself, so why go easy on cancer."

I consoled myself by throwing everything I could find into my arsenal and engaging it as needed except for using food to fight cancer. My reasoning was simple – it seemed like too much work to learn how to cook correctly, and Dr. Harper reported that the tumor appeared to be gone. In fact, my distorted logic caused me to ask why I had to keep taking chemotherapy at all.

By way of answering my question, Dr. Harper explained, "The dose-dense therapy that you are on is extremely rigorous, and most people don't make it through without a break. Would you like to take a break? I'm happy to do that for you, but you'll have to go back on before too long."

"Let me think about that," I said.

I called Suzannah to get her opinion, and she asked me one critical question, "If you take a break, what's the cost?"

"Well, can't I just take the Avastin. Everything I read says it's not as hard to deal with? Then, I can have the surgery followed by radiation. So, I'm not quitting treatment really," I said in a sort of pleading way.

Suzannah patiently explained, "The combination of chemotherapies working together serve as a kind of dishwasher for the body, scrubbing out the far reaches where cancer cells might be hiding. If you just have the mastectomy and parts of the tumor are still present, the surgery could spread cancer to areas it hadn't been before. The radiation is only directed at the areas in close proximity to where the tumor was positioned. So, it's imperative that you finish the chemo and not give the cancer a chance to regain a toe-hold over your body. Think of it this way. You wouldn't stop the dishwasher before it was done with the wash cycle and then eat off those plates, would you?"

I knew she was right. I had to finish the chemo treatments before Dr. Doering could remove my infected breast tissue, so I worked hard to visualize the cancer shriveling up and becoming too weak to metastasize, leaving my bones, lungs, liver and brain free of its "mischief." That's what Dr. Harper called it – mischief. It was a benign term for such a sinister being, but using it seemed like his way of protecting himself from the daily horror of his job. My situation, like so many of his patients, could turn from good to bad in a single day. According to the science, the majority of patients whose cancer recurred did so because the cancer stem cells were resistant to the chemotherapy. That could be true of mine as well, so I marched on and showed up to take my poison. Strangely, I started noticing some odd ball benefits to chemo. My arthritis no longer caused pain; the Morton's neuromas I had developed in my feet after Hannah was born no longer hurt, and the weird bumps on my head disappeared. I was really thankful for that since I didn't have any hair to cover them up. I've heard people talk about good bald and bad bald. Without those bumps, I was in the good bald category, and that just might've been another silver lining.

Ron's brother and his family came to celebrate New Year's with us, but no sooner did they arrive when Ron and Rick moved out on the porch for a night of smoking cigars by the potbelly stove. They smoked and drank almost the entire evening while my sister-in-law Jane and I took care of seven kids. In the interest of my health, she and I decided to accelerate the evening by declaring the New Year's Eve countdown at 10:00 p.m. I changed the clocks in case any of the kids were savvy enough to look, and a few minutes after the hoopla, the house was empty. New Year's Eve on chemo – done.

I put the girls to bed and expected Ron to come in and sit with me, but instead he went out to the deck alone and started a fire in the pit. I watched him from the window with self-pity bantering in my head. I thought he should've been comforting me on the cusp of a new year and was hurt and angry that he wasn't. I caught myself in a self-destructive thought process believing that he truly would be happy if I died. He'd be free to find someone new who was active as I used to be. I stayed at the window long enough to wonder what he was wishing for – a new wife, new home, new town, new friends? It wasn't unheard of for a husband to leave his wife while she battled cancer. Meanwhile, my choices were limited. I was fighting cancer. My life was at best uncertain. I felt isolated and alone. I wanted him to happily hug me, hold me, but instead he treated me as he had treated Sam, our Irish wolfhound, who contracted cancer and slowly declined, dying the spring before I was diagnosed. When Ron banished the ailing dog to the basement, it seemed to me that he just couldn't deal with his own emotions around our impending loss. By contrast, cancer was already growing in my body, but I was unaware of how it was changing everything about me. My emotions ran so high, clouding my ability to understand that what Ron had actually done for Sam was the right thing to do. The dog door was in the basement, so whenever Sam came in from outside, he would try to navigate his gigantic body up the stairs into the rest of the house, but his legs would always give out, leaving him crumpled in a heap at the bottom. By blocking his access to the stairs, Ron had done him a favor, sparing him broken bones and an even earlier demise. To mitigate Sam's loneliness, the girls and I spent hours sitting with him, stroking his massive head and reassuring him that he wasn't alone nor was he separated from his family.

Still clouded by self-pity as I gazed out of my window on the cusp of a new year, I asked myself, "Who would stroke my head?"

I was so tired and scared but remained hopeful for my girls. I was still so alive, so sick and such a burden. Without kids, I probably would've let myself die. Instead, I lived for my girls. While I didn't feel important to Ron, I was to them. So, in the early hours of New Years 2006, I believed for a moment that "in sickness and in health" had flown out of the window.

January 1, 2006
In the morning, the sun rose bright in the sky. What the light of day corrects from the distortion of the dark is incredible. While Ron had been sitting on the deck, he wrote in his journal about how lonely he was. He was more gracious than I had been, however. He was critical of himself for his self-pity when he knew I was suffering in ways he could never know. He wrote that he loved me more than anything, leaving me to feel deeply ashamed for believing he'd be happier without me.

January 5, 2005
While fighting one rare form of aggressive cancer, a second one was lurking undetected in my head and neck. When I was in my early 20's, I had noticed the bump behind my earlobe, and according to my family doctor, it was a gland reacting to the metal in my earrings. Over the years, it came and went never developing into anything major. However, after the mediport was installed, the area grew painful and swollen. At home, I scanned the Susan G. Komen website for anything about IBC moving to the ear lobe and found nothing, so I chalked it up to another side effect and began to cry.

When EmmaGrace saw me, she ordered, "Stop crying, Mommy!"

I felt so bad about upsetting her, and reasoned that even if I only had two to five years of life left, it was better than no years. How I spent those years was up to me, and crying all the time wasn't going to cut it. I could, after all, be in that small percentage of patients that lived more than five years, so I had everything to be happy about. Didn't I? As soon as I talked myself into staying positive, there always seemed to be some new problem that would crop up as if challenging, even testing me with "Are you sure you can stay positive?"

Next up to challenge my emotional state was my chest which felt so heavy, making my breathing more laborious. Positive or not, the fear of lung metastases grew. Dr. Harper must've been slightly concerned as well because he ran me through the MRI machine once again. The results came quickly, and they were negative. While I should've considered clean lungs a victory, I couldn't shake the question of how long would they remain that way, and maybe the cancer just wasn't visible on the scan yet.

January 12, 2005
The fifth chemotherapy was the start of the next phase of treatment, and my body felt the difference. The first pair of chemotherapies left me feeling like lead and painfully toxic with the acrid septic-alcohol aroma permeating my every pore. Hand sanitizer had the same smell, and my doctors insisted that I

use it throughout the day to control the germs around me, but the odor was repulsive. I recoiled whenever my girls thrust a new bottle of scented sanitizer into my nose for a whiff. They were always carrying one or two in their backpacks. No doubt that was a side effect from my/our time in treatment.

In the beginning, Taxol and Avastin didn't make me feel quite as sick, so I tried to settle back into becoming a more involved mom. EmmaGrace was about to lose her first tooth, but her pearly white was holding on despite the emerging adult tooth pushing its way out from underneath. It was several months of tugging, pulling, pushing it out with her tongue, and hanging a camera case off it (EmmaGrace's idea). Nothing we did seemed to work until one day she came home from school buzzing with excitement and thrust her hand into my face so I could get a very up close look at her tooth, bloodied on the end.

She proudly stated, "Look, Mommy! A nice woman with red hair pulled it out for me at school!"

I immediately felt sad and a little cheated. I would've loved to have seen EmmaGrace's face when it finally came out. It was my job to help her, and at the same time, I was grateful to the nice red-haired woman at school, who had lost her mother to breast cancer some years before. I knew she wanted to be helpful, and pulling out the root of EmmaGrace's constant anxiety seemed to do the trick. I turned my attention to what I still had going for me as a mom and made sure the Tooth Fairy was very generous that night.

In the morning, EmmaGrace announced with laughing disbelief, "Mom, the Tooth Fairy left me $5! I know why! Because I had to work so hard to get that tooth out!"

Hannah's language continued to develop during those months. She really didn't say much, but what she did say was perfectly understandable. It was as if she practiced when no one was listening. One day while I lay on the couch in post Neulasta agony, she worked to make me smile by slipping her tiny feet into my Birkenstock sandals sitting next to the couch. Hannah shuffled back and stood in front of me grinning ear to ear.

She declared, "Perfect fit, Mommy. Perfect!"

The girls had no idea how they kept me strong. On one particularly sunny winter's day, I decided to join my family for a walk in the woods behind our house. The unkempt trail led to a small ravine where a fallen poplar tree had created a bridge over the gap. EmmaGrace eyed its broken branches, looking for a path along the trunk to the other side.

"Should I walk over it, Momma?" she asked nervously excited and looking for confirmation that it was safe.

From the log to the bottom of the ravine couldn't have been more than three feet.

I said, "Definitely! You're brave enough."

EmmaGrace walked unsteadily across the log, teetering with her arms outstretched north to south. At the other end, she almost fell off when she celebrated her victory prematurely. Without looking for approval, she ran to the other end and did it over and over.

"You're so brave, Honey!" I cheered.

She responded with a bright smile, "You are too."

Sensing my fatigue building, Ron took my arm and led the girls back to the trail towards home. Energized by her bravery, EmmaGrace ran ahead reaching the house long before we did. When we arrived, Ron opened the door, and inside I could see the table was set and filled in with a very thoughtful spread. EmmaGrace had made a celebratory lunch of ham sandwiches, peeled and cut up carrots, cleaned raspberries and a soda at each place. Sodas were only brought out as a treat for special occasions, and overcoming fears was apparently one such occasion. As I looked closer at the table, a *Sesame Street* song popped into my head, "One of These Things Is Not Like The Others." Sitting at Ron's place was not a soda but an Oktoberfest beer.

"Wow! You did a perfect job! Thank you!" I exclaimed kissing EmmaGrace on the head and giving her a big squeeze.

By cancer treatment standards, it was a perfect day. They weren't always like that. In fact, they were rarely like that, but on that day, I had peace and happiness. It gave me enough of a boost to make another attempt to get back on track and stay focused on my next steps. Instead of living in the present as the cancer counselor's had suggested, I looked ahead because the "present" was full of pain, fear and doubt. I began organizing my thoughts around the anticipated end in July. My modified radical mastectomy was planned for April, followed by 37 radiation treatments, and one more reconstructive surgery, capping off the end of my nightmare. By laying out my benchmarks, I stayed focused on recovery week after week.

January 23, 2006

Before my sixth chemo treatment, Dr. Harper and I discussed what would happen during and after surgery. He told me I'd have to take Herceptin to suppress the hormones so dearly loved by the tumor. I would be on Herceptin for five years, suffering the many side effects that came with it. I didn't like that option, but unfortunately, my weakened cognitive function left me with little ability to come up with any other options. As a way to excuse my growing failure to speak coherently, I often blamed my "chemo brain" likening it to "baby brain." No one really took me seriously until new research started pouring in. My mom cut an article out of the paper announcing a new study, looking at that exact issue. They even called it "chemo brain." I snatched the article from her and held it up as if it was the Holy Grail. The reporter did an excellent job clearly explaining how chemo drugs together with sedatives and steroids caused the release of cytokines, which impaired the brain function of many patients. There it was in black and white, confirming that I was most definitely not going crazy.

Still processing Dr. Harper's Herceptin requirement, I searched for the right words and then blurted out, "Can I have my ovaries removed to cut back on the hormones available to my cancer instead? I don't want to take Herceptin. I also want fewer surgeries, so I want my ovaries removed at the same time as the mastectomy and reconstruction."

Dr. Harper sat back evaluating my requests and their potential ramifications, and then said, "Dr. Doering and Dr. Tousignant have a mutual respect for one another, so I'm sure they would do it. But, you'll have to talk with the plastic surgeon."

He stopped and was quiet for another minute.

Rubbing his chin, he said, "I like it. I think I like that idea a lot. I'll think about it some more and talk with Dr. Doering when I see him next."

"What more can I ask for?" I responded gratefully.

At home, I called Suzannah to talk through the surgery in more detail. Breast cancer and melanoma surgery were her specialties at Memorial Sloan-Kettering, and she was fully equipped to fill in the blanks for me. She explained that during the modified radical mastectomy, I would also have two tiers of lymph nodes removed. Then, if the plastic surgeon agreed to be there, a tissue expander would be implanted followed by Dr. Tousignant performing a laparoscopic bilateral oophorectomy. If all went well, she said, I would only need to follow up with the permanent breast implant surgery sometime in the summer.

Suzannah finished on a high note illuminating the light at the end of the proverbial tunnel, "The oophorectomy and tissue expander are nothing compared to the mastectomy."

Cancer treatment was unrelenting always working to slam down any positive feelings I might be having. The new side effect waiting in the cue was neuropathy. It delivered more suffering as the pain grew in my digits, making it very difficult for me to use my hands. No one could tell me just how long it would last or how painful it would become because every body was different. My fingers were purple and blue, looking as if they had been slammed in a car door. The nails on my index and middle fingers had separated from their nail beds. If I wasn't careful, I could catch them on my clothes, yanking them back as I ejected a blood curdling howl from deep in my core. I couldn't even open the toothpaste tube because the pain was too excruciating. My toes were not spared. They had become numb accompanied by a constant burning sensation, which caused me to walk back on my heels while cursing the medical practitioners that suggested I get out and exercise.

Fortunately, a woman in one of the support groups I rarely attended reported that a hot tub with an ozonating system could reduce the pain and even cure the syndrome. She had gone to a complimentary therapy clinic that provided such a treatment and was elated by the relief. The hot tub on our deck had a similar ozonating system, so I gave it a try. I sat for 45 minutes every day, wishing I had discovered it sooner. It was so peaceful to sit in the warm, aerated water with the cold winter air swirling around me. The bubble of warmth coming off the water's surface surrounded my head like a protective shield, pushing the frigid air just far enough away to keep me comfortable. Every day, my fingers seemed to feel a tiny bit better, and even though it wasn't fast enough, it was moving in the right direction. Today, I've heard from other patients that a simple hot tub produced the same results for them.

January 24, 2006
The impact of Taxol became apparent very quickly. Once again, the side effects of bone pain, body aches and nausea, added to everything else, made it impossible for me to leave the house. On the weekend, Ron's family was celebrating his brother's birthday, and while the tug of family was strong, my body only allowed for one activity each day, and I chose playing with my girls before they left. They were my priority, and that's where I expended my limited energy. In the end, I was so glad I had stayed home because Ron's nana called to speak to me that afternoon.

"How are you feeling? Are you eating? What can I do for you? I'm imagining taking your cheeks in my hands and making you all better," she affectionately said.

83

Her love made me feel warm and cozy through and through, reminding me of my own grandma who had passed in 1993. I paused for a minute, appreciating that Nana was 97 years old and found it within herself to wonder what she could do for me. It was humbling. Since I knew it was important for her to feel needed and her specialty was nurturing through food, I racked my brain for something easy she could make.

Graciously thanking Nana, I said, "I'd love some of your mushroom soup! And, I'm so sorry I'll be missing your party tomorrow."

Even though it was her birthday the next day, Nana was focused on my needs, telling me she'd have the soup delivered as soon as possible. She couldn't really make the soup on her own anymore, so she recruited Aunt Marty to help. I was so appreciative of their love and support, not to mention that wonderful soup, and when it arrived, I drank it in as if it was the elixir of old. Although my taste buds were not yet recovered, I slowly savored the memory of that comforting flavor, feeling loved with every spoon full.

January 25, 2006
Staying at home alone with Hannah was becoming more challenging. She had begun to work on potty training, and while she had mastered urinating on the toilet, her bowels hadn't quite gotten the memo. What was worse was that she wasn't at all bothered by sitting in her dirty diaper, and my compromised olfactory organs didn't pick up the smell until it was thick in the air, saturating the entire house. Continually, I weighed the advice of other parents to either leave a diaper on or put her in regular underwear, but neither one seemed to do the trick. The only difference with the underwear option was that I was far more repulsed and had a much bigger mess to clean up. Trying not to vomit, I would wash Hannah and then, drained from the chore, settle down to watch *Tommy Train* or *Jay Jay Jet Plane* with her. The visions of her bowel movements and the accompanying bacteria stayed with me constantly because of my fear of infection and the increased potential to end up in the hospital as so many other patients had. Seemingly aware that I had performed a disgusting, high-risk chore for her simply because of my unwavering love, a cleaned up Hannah would sing quietly to me or hug me tightly as if wanting me to know how grateful she was.

Sometimes she would even say in response to absolutely nothing, "Love you too, Mommy."

Putting thoughts together was getting harder and harder, and I began to worry about losing what I knew. I imagined it was a little like early Alzheimer's, so I began to write, just to put words down on paper and see if they formed a sentence. I knew I wanted to go back to writing someday, so I poured what little energy I had left into practicing. I was already keeping a journal but wanted some kind of purposeful writing as well. So, I decided to write an email to Ellen DeGeneres. I watched her show during Hannah's nap when I wasn't on the phone and found that it was good for healing and good for my soul. Most days, Ellen was also good for an out loud belly laugh, and I loved her for that. In an odd sort of way, it felt as if she was performing just for me. I never finished the letter because it was too hard for me to write coherently and her producers would've likely tossed it the trash after interpreting my sentiment as that of a crazed fan. Like most things I set my mind to at that time, it faded to gray.

I tried to ignore the pounds coming on fast and furiously because the injustice of it was too hard to comprehend. I had imagined I would be the kind of cancer patient depicted in movies or on television shows, looking so sick and gaunt. I thought losing the last 15 pounds of baby weight was going to be a breeze thanks to cancer treatment and welcomed it as the only tangible perk from my ordeal. So, imagine the deepening chasm of my despair when Dr. Harper confirmed that the steroids I had to take were the culprits helping my body pack on the pounds. It was so unfair. With immediate menopause due to the chemo drugs, lack of exercise, depression and the side effects of prescription medications, my body held on to every pound like a life preserver.

February 6, 2006
I grew weaker and more vulnerable, rarely changing out of my pajamas. My body was much more susceptible to all bacterial or viral infections, which

began to terrify me more than the cancer itself. My resilience was put to the test once again when Hannah brought the stomach flu home from day care. I couldn't be anywhere near her, so I lay in bed weeping, tortured by the sounds of my baby crying out for me. Although I knew Ron was taking good care of her, I grabbed a damp rag from my bathroom to put over my nose and mouth before going to her bedroom in hopes of relieving her anguish. I wanted her to know I hadn't abandoned her.

"I'm sorry I can't hold you, Honey. You've got the flu, and I can't get sick, or I could end up in the hospital. I love you and want you to feel better!" I said blowing her a weak kiss before stumbling back to bed.

My chest was feeling the cumulative effects of chemo. It was very heavy and hurt constantly, causing me to fall prey to the fear that cancer was spreading, spreading and spreading some more. For some reason, a flood of comments others had spoken to me during my challenge took over my thoughts that night. I delved in to over analyzing every shred of advice. The words "Put your faith in God" were so often spoken, but I started to question how praying was going to help me get through each challenge. Relinquishing control, "Let Go. Let God" felt passive. Was I helpless? I wondered if letting go was just a coping mechanism like saying "I put my life in God's hands," so if I die, it's on Him. Did it mean I was giving up? I didn't want to give up. Then it hit me. All of those words of advice were pushing me to continue to find and engage the resources God had provided. Lying in bed, I prayed for victory. I prayed to be patient and calm. I prayed to be alive in 40 years. I prayed to stay on the path God had created for me. I prayed my kids wouldn't suffer any more trauma in their lives. Bumps in the road were okay, but no real trauma like me dying. I lay there with every healthy cell in my body exhausted, and intentionally choosing to take the advice I had been given, I took a breath in, then let go and let God and fell asleep.

Exploration

February 13, 2006

"The only thing that makes life possible is permanent, intolerable uncertainty: not knowing what comes next." –Ursula K. Le Guin

As I lay on the pea green couch trying to meditate as I did every day, I was alone in the house staring out the window and watching the clouds when a blanket of pure peace spread out over me. I felt it. I physically felt the warmth melt the stress and worry away. I had no other explanation than to believe that it was God calling me home. I was going to die, and it felt right. I was completely at peace with it. I mentally ran through whether or not my affairs were in order and who would help Ron be a parent. I made one final prayer that my girls would always know happiness, safety and love, closed my eyes and drifted off to sleep in a blissful state, believing I would never wake up. However, my expiration was obviously not yet part of THE plan because I woke to the sound of the front door slamming and heard a sweet little voice call me, "Mommy!" I giggled at my melodrama. It wasn't my time. God was just letting me feel His arms around me. The peace I felt was truly the peace of knowing everything was going to be all right.

Ron yelled as he walked through the door with his arms full, "Can you get Hannah? She has to go potty?"

I jumped up without a second to spare, swept her up in my arms and sped her to the bathroom. Instead of forcing the happy, positive tone around how exciting it was to be a big girl using the potty, I felt sincere in my elation, and she joined in. Instead of looking nervous to be on the toilet, Hannah let loose the moment I sat her down. When she was all done, she gave me a huge grin. I cheered; she cheered; Ron cheered from the kitchen, and Hannah and I washed our hands. That was, of course, her favorite part. She loved the bubbly suds all over her skin. While she rinsed the soap off, I laughed again at myself and thought about how powerful life was.

During my seventh chemo infusion, I was watching television when a commercial for St. Jude's Children's Hospital came on. I burst into inconsolable sobbing. I cried so hard I could barely breathe. How could those sweet little faces be subjected to this same agony? Were my girls at higher risk because of my diagnosis? It used to be that childhood cancer was rare, but in 2015, every day would see 45 American children being diagnosed. It was absolutely criminal. It was also true that prior to 1980, it was very rare for a child to be diagnosed with type 2-diabetes; however, by 2014, the number of children diagnosed in my home state of Wisconsin continued to grow. The World Health Organization estimated that 60% of the world population would suffer some sort of chronic illness such as cancer, obesity, diabetes, or heart disease by the year 2020, and it was no secret that those diseases could be linked to the poor quality of our food and the environment. Obesity, diabetes and heart disease were all risk factors for cancer and had some relationship to food. According to the National Cancer Institute, 39% of U.S. citizens would be diagnosed with cancer at some point in their lives, and more than 14 million currently lived with it. I just couldn't understand why public health, safety and ultimately the economy as a whole were pushed to the side in favor of individual corporate profits. How could economic development in this country succeed with the ever-increasing costs of health care causing so many to file for personal bankruptcy? Allowing insurance and drug companies to reap excessive profits from chronic disease didn't seem like an economically sustainable system for a world super power. From what I was reading, the U.S. was the only country in the developed world not negotiating lower prices with the pharmaceutical industry. When I fired my ramblings out to the care givers around me at my appointments, I wasn't really asking anyone to respond because I already knew they agreed.

At my next appointment, Dr. Harper entered the room, and I posed one of my policy questions to him. Not wanting to go down that rabbit hole with me, he masterfully switched the topic of discussion to praising me for not taking a break from my treatment. Since I had "soldiered" on, he believed the consistent attack on the cancer would greatly reduce its ability to recur. Happily, his comments trumped the sadness I felt about the out of control chronic disease in our world, and instead of crying, I was elated.

Nurse Judy and Dr. Harper sent me on my way with these words, "It's not hard to look around and find someone worse off."

It was a true statement, but relatively speaking, I was worse off than anyone I knew at the time. So, while it was true, it wasn't helpful. Cancer was not so much of a journey for me, but a ride on the world's most emotional roller coaster. It started with a few dips to build momentum, then sped me on my way into treatment, followed by a long slog uphill with the death-defying flips and twists of side effects and finally a slow coast back to a new state of health and being, stripping me of everything I knew. When I was first diagnosed, I became angry, then focused, followed by emotional, exhausted, hopeful, exhausted, taxed, angry, exhausted, focused, etc. The whole experience forced me to rewrite my story, change my habits and behaviors, and step away from who I was in order to become who I was meant to be.

I bought the *Anti-Cancer* book by David Servan-Schreiber, MD, and *Foods That Fight Cancer* by Richard Belliveau and began to study their work. Eventually, the *Anti-Cancer* book became a bible of sorts for me. I read it over and over so carefully and slowly, that it seemed every word was etched on each cell in my body. It was one of the few books that was easy for me to read at the time, and I placed it prominently on the kitchen counter to refer to whenever I forgot what I needed to know, which was often. I referred to the chart Dr. Servan-Schreiber provided on cancer fighting foods and tried to eat as many as I could every day. His list wasn't very different from the one I was already using, but it had pictures. He cited research that was showing how cancer stem cells resistant to chemotherapy were vulnerable to anti-angiogenic foods, and since I ate food throughout the day, I needed to make it count. I finally forced myself into a completely anti-angiogenic diet and imagined every bite was an ax chopping away at the tumor's blood supply as if chopping down a tree. Food would become my medicine, and for a self-professed foodie, what could be better.

"Let food be thy medicine and medicine be thy food." – Socrates.

It wasn't long before it became easier to follow my plan to eat food as medicine. Every day, I committed to eating 10 items from my list. Some days, it was nearly impossible, but I sat at the table anyway with my head resting on my arm determined to take little bites of cabbage, leeks, sweet potatoes, collard greens, Swiss chard, Brussel sprouts, strawberries and blueberries among others until my plate was empty. Sometimes, I would sit there for a full hour just to get it all in. I looked at food as another form of chemo, but one that wouldn't have nasty side effects and would feed my recovery without severe damage to my body. The list of foods I settled on was a conglomeration of a list from a variety of sources including the *Anti-Cancer* book and food science researchers I had met along the way. I took copious notes during my phone conversations, synthesizing them later at my much slower pace. Eating with the intention to heal gave me something positive to pivot on and seemed to begin to wake up my brain cells. Food science researcher Dr. Gary Stoner welcomed me into his world-renowned berry lab housed in the Wisconsin Medical College. His research focused primarily on the cancer-fighting properties of black raspberries and strawberries with incredible results. I was grateful to all the scientists who embraced my will to live. Knowing them made me feel as if I was part of something bigger.

February 16, 2006
With my last chemo treatment around the corner, I met with Dr. Doering to

discuss my upcoming mastectomy.

"Depending on what I find when I perform the mastectomy, you may need more chemo," he said, looking straight into my eyes with that familiar compassion.

He explained the grenade-shaped rubber balls that would hang from tubes stitched under my skin at the mastectomy site. Pinned to my shirt, they would collect the fluid draining from my body, instead of letting it build up, which could cause a variety of physical complications.

"On a positive note, I spoke with Dr. Sanders, and he has agreed to tag team the surgery with us. Isn't that great! You'll have a plastic surgeon right there to close the wounds," he said, working so hard to find the bright spot in all of it for me.

Having all three surgeons working on me at essentially the same time really was a bright spot. I had scored a major coup over the medical system, which meant I would go under anesthesia one time not three. I would only endure the risks of surgery and its difficulties once. I would only have the staggering costs of surgery once. I was elated. One and done! The mastectomy, oophorectomy and placement of the tissue expander would all be completed on April 6, 2006. After that, I would have one more surgery to replace the tissue expander with a breast implant, and then I could finally start to move on from cancer, or so I thought.

In preparation for my surgical coup, Dr. Tousignant explained that my insurance company would only cover one night in the hospital.

"You'll have to go home the day after surgery unless," she paused, "you develop a terrible headache, nausea or some other post-surgical problem."

She gave me a wink, and I immediately understood her meaning. It was true. Most insurance companies would not allow a woman having a breast amputated to remain in the hospital for more than one night, which I found simply outrageous. While I couldn't fully understand the pain and agony I would feel, I could imagine it. My time with cancer really put a magnifying

glass on the massive faults in our health care system, but luckily, my doctors went the extra mile to navigate around them. The injustice and lack of respect shown to those who suffer most was unconscionable. I couldn't understand how my government had gotten so far afield that corporate profits superseded the priority of public health.

February 24, 2006

My last chemotherapy came on the heels of Ron's brother's wedding in Chicago. It was by far the toughest weekend and was compounded by the assignment of my daughters to be flower girls, which meant I had to "work." It felt like an impossible task since I spent most of my time horizontal. Measurements for their dresses began in the months leading up to the wedding, but because of my compromised eyesight, I could hardly make out the tiny numbers on the tape measure. Luckily, Aunt Marty came to my rescue and completed the task.

The rehearsal was on a Friday afternoon at St. Pauls United Church in Chicago built in 1855. Since my brother's party, I hadn't driven more than 30 minutes from my house, and a drive to Chicago was tough to wrap my head around. So, pushing the growing anxiety aside with a couple of Lorazepam tablets, I dressed in my most comfortable elastic waistband pants, collapsed into the front seat, popped my ear buds in to stream meditation music, closed my eyes and settled in for the grueling three-hours of stop-and-go traffic. Happily, the combination did the trick, granting me sleep the entire way, and I only woke up when Ron pulled up in front of the brick church. He parked in front of its wide open, massive, quadruple wooden doors, beckoning us to enter under an arched stained-glass window. Through the vestibule was another set of carved wooden doors so heavy I struggled to pull them open. Oozing reverence, I ushered the girls into the main chapel where the pews were separated from an open hall. Both sides were lined with stone archways capped by white walls, holding a series of bowed stained glass windows. Each intricately colorful window told a different part of Jesus' life and His ascension into heaven. Still foggy with sleep, I stumbled along with the girls through the church into a room on the other side of the wall. It was there that I found my momentary salvation. My sister-in-law Amy graciously offered to spare me the confusion of trying to figure out what the girls were supposed to do and directed me to follow her lead. Miraculously, none of us made a mistake, at least not one that Amy told me about, and when our tasks were concluded, I promptly sunk into the last pew in the chapel and closed my eyes, fighting the urge to lie down.

As if the following day wasn't exciting enough for the girls, I had to go and send them over the moon by foolishly taking them to the Shedd Aquarium on Lake Michigan. Ron worried that I wouldn't be able to walk through the exhibits, and, to be honest, so was I. Just thinking about it wore me down. We took what was the girls' first cab ride, and their unbridled enthusiasm elicited a clear annoyance from the driver. I laughed quietly to myself as they narrated everything they saw between the hotel and aquarium. Relieved to finally eject us from his cab, the driver stoically dropped us at the bottom of the steps leading to the entrance, took his cash and sped off without a word. As always,

I shuffled along behind the girls using Ron's arm for support as he dragged me up the stairs to the ticket window. Inside the building, I scoped out benches here and there, stealing a rest at each one while Ron trailed the girls through the exhibits. In the afternoon, we watched the beluga whale show, and a s much as I was against supporting the practice of keeping whales in captivity, I gratefully attended because it offered me respite for 30 continuous minutes with not one single thing to do. As soon as my fanny hit the chair, my eyes closed automatically, and I listened happily to the girls shriek with delight as the belugas performed their tricks. *(Just so you know, I winced as I wrote those words, because no wildlife should perform tricks for any humans.)*

Back at the hotel, we began the arduous task of getting both girls bathed, dressed and attempted to arrange their hair in the requisite style before the 5:00 p.m. wedding ceremony. Ron was my only help because amidst the excitement of wedding mayhem, my handicap was forgotten. He fumed with silent anger as I cried. Admittedly, my sadness and depressive emotions were always right at the surface quick to break through with the slightest ripple, and that day was no exception. I was so exhausted that my eyes closed uncontrollably as I cried. Ron picked up the pieces once again and took over styling the girls' hair, but neither of us did a very good job, so I asked Ron to get help. Without a word, he left the room to track someone down, but in an instant I knew I had made a mistake. I should've recognized how frustrated he was because through the closed door I heard an explosion in the hall.

"None of you have any idea what Kathy is going through and how hard this weekend is for her!"

He stormed back into our room, slammed the door and started to brush EmmaGrace's hair. We quietly did our best with the girls, and I donned my wig. That was all we could do. I made it through the ceremony and kept the girls calm until after the pictures and then relinquished my duties to the babysitters that were employed to entertain the smaller children in a room separate from the reception. EmmaGrace and Hannah were so excited to play with kids their own age, and when we arrived at the door, they whizzed right past us without even looking back. The happy chaos had already begun, and that sure beat staying with their mom any longer than necessary. During the reception, I stayed close to Ron as he chatted with friends and relatives. I smiled here and there but was always on the lookout for a corner to sit in.

Unable to follow the conversations, I wandered off, but before I was out of earshot I heard Ron's uncle say, "Ronny, she looks really good."

Ron responded, "She's really good at faking it."

I slipped out and made my way up to where the kids were. It was pure joyful chaos. The babysitters chased after kids running into the halls of the historic hotel, but somehow no one noticed me parked on a bench outside of the room. I watched the evening tick on until I couldn't sit up any more, almost an hour had passed before I collected the girls, and we all went to bed. I survived. That's how difficult the weekend was for me. There was no enjoyment, just survival, and when we got home on Sunday, I had to prepare for my last day of poisoning.

"I am the Toxic Avenger," I said out loud and then let out a little giggle before going to sleep.

February 27, 2006
The exhaustion from the weekend fell away, making room for my elation with the last day of chemo.

When Ron and the girls dropped me off, I cheered, "Yea, last chemo day!"

EG cheered, "Yippee! Now you just have to get your boob chopped off!"

I smiled at her and gave her a quick peck, "That's one way to look at it. Have a fun day."

I arrived at the cancer center, submitted to the requisite blood draw and was escorted to the toxic chamber they called a treatment room. I smiled and chatted until the sedative took hold, sending me into a drowsy, relaxed state for the rest of the day. When my nurse came in to pull the infusion needle out, I let loose a sleepy cheer, which was trumped by the cancer center staff appearing in my room with a package of gifts to celebrate the end. It included a certificate of achievement, an angel pin and a glass heart etched with the word "Hope." I felt a little embarrassed when I held that heart because I hadn't really lived in hope. Throughout my treatment I prayed for strength and determination. Had I prayed around hope, I may have found despair. So, hope felt sad to me until one of the cancer counselors explained to me that I had engaged hope when I wisely embraced all that God had offered me. I also questioned my team when they cheered me as a survivor. I didn't feel like a victim of cancer, so how could I be a survivor? The evolution of my ideas about the diagnosis were evolving into being more of a learning opportunity for me. With the help of several people in my life, I used all of the resources God had given me, including my ability to question, challenge and suggest that no stone be left unturned and no weapon left idle. In the end, if the cancer won, so be it, but I knew it wouldn't. My team was stronger. My team had God, love, science, technology, knowledge, skill, compassion and tenacity.

93

Ron wore the pink *"YMe"* bracelet given out at the cancer center every day during my treatment. He picked one up for me too, but I couldn't wear it. It made me feel too much like a victim. I wasn't going to wear a question of weakness on my wrist because it was a question I couldn't afford to ask. There was too much wallowing in that phrase, but he wanted to outwardly show his undying support for me and wouldn't take it off until I was done.

When he arrived to pick me up with Hannah, I grabbed his arm and snatched off the bracelet.

"I'm done. Now, get rid of this thing," I demanded.

He quickly obliged.

Unfortunately, the elated energy of the end didn't follow me home. I was dog-tired and ornery as always. It felt as if I was in a dream. I couldn't believe I was done with cancer and all that was left was the cleanup. Thank God, I couldn't see what was to come.

Two hours after finishing my last chemo, I lay in bed at home thinking about the climbers who reached the summit of Mount Kilimanjaro and how they might toss off their gear and open their arms to the space of their success. I needed a release like that, but instead of joy, everything I had carried on the way up to the chemo summit came pouring out in an uncontrollable wailing and river of tears. Through it all, I could still hear EmmaGrace in the hall counting her allowance out loud as she dropped it into the toy ATM bank with a digital screen tallying her loot. I gave up a little laugh, and soon I couldn't tell if I was crying from happiness or sadness. That little break jettisoned my attention onto more positive thoughts. The first thing I was most looking forward to after that chemotherapy was getting off Coumadin. I had been previously diagnosed with antiphospholipid syndrome, a blood clotting disorder, so Coumadin or Lovonox were the drugs of choice to help me avoid a blood clot. I preferred Coumadin because it was a pill as opposed to Lovonx, which was a shot in the stomach every day. During my pregnancy with Hannah, I had taken it, and it was awful. I irrationally worried the needle would go too deep and I would pierce my baby. Blood thinners were a stressful medication because added to the frailty of my body was the potential risk of bleeding to death. Gratefully, I could finally release that anxiety and focus on restoring my physical strength.

That last treatment hit me like a ton of bricks, and I slept for two days solid. At the end of the week, I heard from one of our family members who asked, "Do you feel better now that you've had almost a week to rest?"

It was said with sincerity and compassion, but utter ignorance of what "chemo week" really was. I knew it was hard to know what to say to someone going through what I was because every once in a while, I'd say the wrong thing to someone and just cringe at myself. In the beginning, those kinds of comments were offensive to me, but after all of the meditation and prayer occupying the majority of my waking hours, I had developed a more compassionate reaction that permitted me to respond graciously. Unfortunately, I still hadn't learned how to extend that same courtesy to myself. My fragile emotional state was front and center every single day. I cried inconsolably as I took stock of my physical state. My mouth tasted like metal. The anti-nausea medication, Zofran, gave me intense headaches. My fingers were painful, purple and quite scary-looking since I had been neglecting my hot tub treatments. My breathing had become harder, and my nose was raw and bloody, having lost all of its hair. I lost my eyebrows and eyelashes, which might not seem like a big deal, but it really changed my appearance even more than a bald head had. I became much more self-conscious in public, and so I rarely left the house.

By Sunday, I was able to drag myself out to the barn with Ron's help. EmmaGrace brushed the horses while he and Hannah filled the water tank outside the barn door. Slowly, I picked the poop and dirty shavings out of the stalls, and when I was done, Ron held my arm as I plodded along back to the house. We changed into our swimming suits and settled in for a much-deserved family soak in the hot tub. I let the ozonized water quell the painful effects of neuropathy, and took in long, deep breaths, letting the warmth of the tub go to work on my bedraggled body.

EmmaGrace stared at me for a long minute and said, "Mommy, I'm afraid you're going to lose to cancer."

I was absolutely heartbroken and had nothing to say.

"I know Mommy looks pretty bad right now, but that's because she's getting better," Ron said trying to explain the paradox of chemotherapy. "If you think Mom looks bad, think about the cancer. It's just a broken jumbled mess being carried out of Mom's body every time she goes number two."

Even I laughed at the visual of mortally wounded cancer cells trapped in the sludge of my excrement. Leave it to Ron to successfully take our "hot-tub-hang-out-conversation" in a much more entertaining direction.

95

March 2006

EmmaGrace was becoming more comfortable talking about where I was in my recovery and started to ask questions I didn't know how to answer.

"What if one cancer cell survives? Will you get cancer again and die?" my second grader inquired.

I had no idea how to answer her, and in my discomfort blurted out, "I won't get cancer again. We are doing everything we can to kill every last cell. I'm really strong, Honey, and nothing is going to take me away from you."

It was clearly written on her face that something wasn't resonating for her, and it made me feel so sad that she was worried. She was just too young to have fears like that. She knew I was lying because I was always worried about the cancer lurking in some other part of my body, growing resistant to the toxic soup I had endured.

I asked her what else she wanted to ask, and she said, "Some kids at school said you're probably going to die."

That statement knocked me down onto one of the wooden chairs in the kitchen. I wondered how a second grader would even know that was a possibility, but then I realized they must've heard it from their parents. I was horrified. It was already such a huge burden for EmmaGrace to live with a parent battling cancer, but the rumors circulating through school and making their way back to her gave her nowhere left to find solace. School had been her happy place, her safe place. She didn't have to look at me, watch me or hear me. Up until that insensitive statement from the boys, EmmaGrace had all but forgotten her upside down life at home. I couldn't stop the tears from welling up in my eyes.

"Don't cry, Mama. I don't like it," EmmaGrace ordered and then walked away.

Once the news of my last chemo was out, the phone calls began pouring in. It seemed the war had ended. The last bugle call pledging to guard and honor the fallen was over. The moment of silence had been lifted, and morning had broken. With each phone call, I spoke positive words with strength to match the enthusiasm on the other end.

"It's gone. We beat it. We hit it with everything, but…my surgery will tell more of the story. The doctors feel good about it, and so do I," I asserted with as much confidence as I could muster, hoping I'd believe it too.

I thought of it as the power of suggestion, but after hanging up with each call, I slumped in the chair from the weight of my act. I didn't feel strong, but I couldn't let on. It would only illicit sympathy followed by uncomfortable silences, and as long as I stayed positive, everyone was happy. I could feel in control for just a brief moment, resisting the fear of never really knowing for sure.

Dr. Harper called to let me know he had followed up with the oncologists at the National Institute of Health and Memorial Sloan-Kettering who confirmed that there was no further chemotherapy treatment option for me except to add Tamoxifen on top of my impending surgeries and radiation. I had wished I could've been in on those conversations because I was a big picture person and wanted to know all about the potential twists and turns in my story so I could react quickly and waste no time, if indeed they happened. The stress of it all was manifesting itself in terrible headaches, and Dr. Harper took them more seriously than I did. He sent me in for a brain MRI to look for the potential cause, which was code for another tumor or metastases. I welcomed his attention to reducing my stress and found peace of mind in knowing nothing was growing. However, the constant stress fed my crabby attitude, which did not go unnoticed by my seven-year-old.

"Momma, why are you always so crabby?" EmmaGrace asked with a slight sting in her words.

I didn't want to answer it how I did, but my energy was so depleted that I could only give her the words true to my heart. It was important for her to know how stressful my situation was, but I didn't want her to feel as if any of it was her fault. I truly was conflicted because the concept seemed too much for her tender age.

"This is the hardest thing I've ever done, Peanut. Even though I know I'm strong enough to beat the cancer, it's always in the back of my mind that I might be wrong. It's natural to be afraid even though I believe I'll be OK. When the fear creeps in, it brings a lot of stress with it, and sometimes I struggle to control my outbursts. I'm so sorry. Daddy is also stressed because he's been doing my job, his job and taking care of me on top of it. He's very tired and worried the cancer could win, but I'm not going to let that happen. You can help us out big time by not arguing when things don't go your way. We're a team and need to stick together. I've never been good at letting people take care of me because I like to take care of everyone else, but this time I really do need your help. I need everyone working to get me better so that our life can go back to normal and be fun again. Remember, we are three brave women…and one brave man," I assured her with a hug.

"Can we talk about something else?" she asked.

"Of course! What would you like to talk about?"

"There's a boy named Patrick that I think is really nice," she said ending our conversation by skipping off to play.

I never had any idea what was the right thing to tell her. I'm not sure anyone knew the best way to talk to kids about cancer, but as a parent, I tried to do what I could and hoped for the best.

Every little ache and pain continued to loom larger than life even though I practiced meditation every day. I had terrible night sweats. The toes on my right foot were numb, and the nails on five fingers had pulled away and died. The other ones yellowed but were still attached. I worried about infections constantly. My skin was thinner and would split fairly easily. Piled on top of that, were the symptoms of menopause, which I had entered after the first chemo treatment, but no one prepared me for what to expect, so the hot flashes took me by surprise. My body temperature jumped from hot to cold then hot back to cold. It was nonstop throughout the day and night. Why would I be spared that additional discomfort just because I had cancer and suffered so much already? The answer was, I wouldn't. It was getting harder to face the reality of being someone with chronic pain, but there was no other way to characterize it.

Overall, I lived in continuous discomfort. I needed more oxygen and exercise but was too exhausted to grab it. When I tried, it took everything I had and left nothing for the girls. My stomach hurt all the time, but I wasn't sure if it was hunger pains or nausea caused by the drainage from my bloody nose. My back, eyes and head hurt, and every bone ached. I couldn't seem to find relief anywhere except during drug-induced sleep. Positive thinking eluded me often, and my thoughts drifted towards the end and how much easier it would be if I had died. Even though I pushed them out as soon as they took hold in my mind, sometimes they lingered, bringing a muted smile to my face. Somehow I found peace in the thought of quitting, even though it was absolutely out of the question. Instead I looked for ways to keep myself from falling too deeply into that bottomless pit of depression and settled on carrying a small photo album with pictures of my girls. Re-evaluating my discomfort, I found that my tongue no longer hurt as much, and my hair was starting to grow. It was no longer blonde, and the curls were gone, but I was excited to see the peach fuzz covering my scalp no matter what it looked like. My nurse Judy told me it would grow about half an inch each month, which gave me another reason to smile. At one appointment, Dr. Harper asked if he could feel my hair. He really liked the feel of new hair. I should've asked him why but lacked the energy. I wondered if it represented a potential victory or was just a tactile perk for him since he dealt with death on a weekly basis. His reason didn't matter; however, because he had earned the right to touch my new hair.

When Dr. Harper and I discussed my physical state, I primarily focused on menopause. When it came on, I felt as if I was trapped in a 200-degree sauna, and nothing worked to cool me down. Then came the nausea and light headedness, which ushered in yet another medication. It was his opinion that it was time to start an anti-depressant called Zoloft. He explained that it would help my mood and had the off-label benefit of "quieting" menopausal symptoms. I raced to the pharmacy and picked up the newest addition to my medicine chest and popped one in my mouth right at the check-out counter. With my own chaotic bedside pharmacy, I often forgot which drugs did what, which could've been disastrous since I was convinced I needed each and every one of them throughout the day. I was certain my doctors wouldn't have prescribed them if I didn't need them, so I mixed and matched looking for relief because no one said I shouldn't.

After a few weeks, Dr. Harper followed up to see how I was doing after starting Zoloft. I wasn't sure how to answer him since I still felt anxious, but it seemed to stay inside instead of exploding out. I asked him if it would eventually go away all together, but he didn't have an answer for me and suggested I see a counselor. He felt that the fear and anxiety, while normal, were maybe the hardest part of a cancer diagnosis. In all honesty, it didn't make any sense to me that I would be depressed. I was in remission after all. How could I possibly be depressed? Was I sad that the circled wagons had dispersed? Was it that I had more free time to assess my situation and the grave nature of my diagnosis was finally clear? Was it another side effect of the drugs? No one could tell me, and I guess it didn't really matter. The truth was that depression had invaded my space, and I had to deal with it.

In an effort to lighten my load, Dr. Harper said, "You're going to make it. You're going to be all right."

The following morning Hannah asked her first "why" question, "Why do we sit on chairs?"

I answered, "So we don't fall and get hurt."

She said, "OK."

99

I wished the answers I was seeking were so easily found. I scheduled another lunch with my friends in an effort to drag myself out of the house and focus on something other than my growing anxiety and depression disorders, but once again, our lunch was thwarted with both of my girls coming down with pink eye.

As a result, I developed a sore throat and cough and resigned myself to another week at home.

I threw away another year, announcing very loudly, "2007 will be a better year for all of us!"

March 25, 2006
For my 42nd birthday Ron, had organized a ski trip to Colorado, and I was all in. It was another decision that seemed almost comical as I looked back at what I thought I could do. Of all the natural landscapes, I loved the mountains most. I pulled out my green suitcase, tossed it on my bed and unzipped the main pocket. I folded up my polar fleece long underwear, leggings that fit under my ski pants, polar fleece tops, wool sweaters and elastic waist band pants, placing them in a pile on my bed. I turned my attention to my daily medicines, which sent my mind to the specter of myriad viral and bacterial organisms surrounding me at the airport. It was a minefield void of safety, and I could only protect myself if I had a plethora of options. So, I packed as if traveling required a germ warfare survival kit of sorts. I filled a gallon-sized Ziplock bag with prescription medications and a variety of herbal remedies that I had read about in one of the many books I had been given. I packed chaparral, astragalus, marshmallow root, echinacea, goldenseal, rosehips, peppermint, chamomile, vitamin C, zinc, probiotics and Lansinoh to slather in my nasal passages. Even though it was designed to help breast-feeding mothers heal their painful, chapped nipples, Lansinoh seemed to be working in my nostrils, and I reasoned that its viscous properties doubled as a trap to catch any organisms attempting to penetrate my body via my nose. I loved traveling when I was healthy, but the fear of what could go wrong now overwhelmed any enthusiasm I had mustered.

While the flight was uneventful, entering our rented condominium was not. My chest tightened, and my hands started to shake as my eyes darted from space to space, scanning the floors and corners of each room for dirt and studying the upholstery on each piece of furniture for stains. The sounds from the movie *Psycho* played over and over in my head, and tears poured from my eyes. Catching me before I went too far, Ron swept me up and led me to our room to adjust my reality before I ruined the happy moment our girls so badly deserved. They ran throughout the place leaving a trail of blankets, stuffed animals and

APRIL 1, 2006

The minute we got home, I was mercilessly thrown back into scanning and preparing for surgery. MRI and PET scans brought a level of comfort nothing else could've at that time, but waiting for the results was a real nail biter. Would they still see cancer where it had been? Would they see it somewhere else? Would it really be gone if they didn't see it at all? Two of my three questions were answered when the radiologist gave me the "all clear," and my doctors officially labeled me in remission and ready for surgery. However, they were unwilling to say that the cancer was completely gone because the odds were they'd see it on the next set of scans. For me, it would have to be enough for the time being.

While I searched for joy, my emotions were tempered with the understanding that an "all clear" could really mean "nothing was visible at that moment," which was punctuated by a new problem brewing in my lungs. My breathing had become labored, and of course, my go to culprit was cancer. Even though no cancer activity was picked up by my scans, it was more than possible that those tiny invaders had penetrated my lung tissue undetected. It wouldn't have been the first time scans had missed those evil little scoundrels.

"Let's not jump to the worst case scenario first," Dr. Harper said encouraging me. "I want to check how your lungs are working."

He knew better than to only see my symptoms through the prism of metastasized cancer and sent me for a pulmonary function test to assess how well my lungs were sending oxygen into my blood and whether or not I was suffering from lung toxicity, another side effect of treatment. The results supported his theory and showed my lung capacity had significantly decreased, but it was just high enough that surgery was still a go. Dr. Harper was happy, but for me it was still a lot of missing oxygen, especially when the impending radiation therapies were likely to reduce it even more. While I was relieved, the prospect of recurrence was only pushed to the back of my mind not obliterated all together.

Since Zoloft seemed to finally be doing its job, the news of my damaged lungs was easier to take. I had fewer hot flashes and felt less anxious. Ron, on the other hand, seemed to be having trouble keeping it together. More often than not, he was crabby and yelled at the girls over the littlest things.

"I think you should take something," I coaxed.

"I spent my entire adolescence on drugs and I'm not going there again. I become an addict quickly, so I'm staying away," he responded with a note of venomous helplessness.

Suzannah suggested a support group for spouses. It was a great idea, so I called Stillwaters Cancer Support Services, a non-profit organization co-founded by Dr. Harper. I gave Ron the dates and times of the group meetings and he pledged to try and make it work but never did. He was too reserved to emote with complete strangers. My mom subtly gave him a life line not long after. While standing together on the pool deck at the YMCA watching Hannah in her swim class, my mom gave him a pocket crucifix.

"Whenever I feel anxious, I touch it. I find it gives me that little bit of comfort I need," she whispered.

I was entirely surprised that he embraced her gift, especially since he often professed to be an atheist. Perhaps all he needed was a little nudge towards faith. He slipped it in his pocket and whispered thank you.

I anxiously drafted contingency plans around my recovery from surgery and slipped from my meditation practice, rendering peace elusive once again. As the date of surgery grew closer, I specifically developed nervous energy around the modified radical mastectomy. I peppered my doctors with questions from my growing list, but they didn't understand that I needed to wrap my head around what they were going to do to me. I instead of answering me in any meaningful way, they gave me abbreviated answers followed by suggestions that I not look at any surgical videos online. So I gave up pressing and went to my back-up plan – Suzannah. I asked her the same probing questions, but all she would say was that Dr. Doering had done many surgeries like it and knew exactly what he was doing. Recognizing my lack of satisfaction with her answer, Suzannah reluctantly continued with a brief explanation of what they would be looking for.

"Dr. Doering will be removing as much breast tissue as he can from your right side along with the lymph nodes laying under your armpit. He'll ask the pathologist to look at the sentinel nodes, the ones that are first off the breast tissue, to see if any cancer has made its way into them. He won't be able to get all of the breast tissue. No one can. So, there is always some left on the chest wall. As a result, your risk of recurrence will not be 0%. Once he's done his part, Dr. Sanders will insert a tissue expander and close up your wound. It will be a big scar, so don't be surprised by that. Dr. Tousignant's part is quick. She will go in laparoscopically and remove your ovaries, leaving a tiny scar that you'll never really notice once it's healed. After that, you'll go home and manage the drains for a couple of weeks, but don't make the mistake of doing more than the doctors allow. If you do too much, you'll likely have the drains in longer."

Suzannah and I talked about the benefits of having a double mastectomy instead. It would be easier to get matching breasts in reconstruction and would alleviate some of the risk of cancer spreading to my left side. However, amputating just one breast was difficult enough let alone two. At the time, there was no clear research pointing to the actual benefits of a double amputation and she felt very strongly that I should just do the infected side. I took her comments to Dr. Harper who agreed, and I tried to convince myself that in a year's time, it would seem like a pointless debate. I anticipated that the plastic surgeon would give me perky boobs and I'd be free to go on my merry way. Ten years later, however, I think I should've opted for the double, just for the aesthetics. Because no matter how many surgeries I've had, my breasts have never looked anywhere near the same.

The next debilitating side effect came out of the blue, making any and all noise deafening in my head. It didn't matter if I was by myself or in a room with others chattering away. I couldn't take the noise.

When the girls spoke to me I desperately pleaded, "Not now. I need quiet in my head!"

Then, I would shuffle off to my room and shut the door. On one such day, I decided to get back to meditating and hit play on my Ipod, which sent soothing meditation melodies through my ears but even that was too much. I turned it off and lay quietly, listening to my breath before drifting into a peaceful slumber. When I woke, I jumped for joy with the understanding that I could meditate without music. It was a game changer for me. I would no longer be encumbered by an Ipod. My mind shifted to looking forward to my hospital stay. It would be two full days during which I wouldn't have to think about anyone but myself. Two full days of being cared for. Two full days of relative silence.

EmmaGrace asked again if I could get cancer more than once. Unfortunately, I gave her the wrong answer.

"No, we got it all. I shouldn't have it again."

Then I pleaded with God, "Please, God. Not again."

APRIL 5, 2006
The morning of my surgery went very smoothly. When we dropped EmmaGrace off at school, I gave her a huge hug and kiss. She raced through

the doors without ever looking back. Then, at Ron's parents, I held Hannah tight before leaving her, telling her I'd be home soon. During the drive to the hospital, I sat quietly processing the consensual maiming that was about to occur. My parents met us there and I dug deep for a smile. By that time, I really appreciated disappearing into my own silence and spoke very little. In the pre-operation room, I disrobed, dressed in the hospital gown and lay still while the nurses ran through a battery of questions before inserting the IV needle through which they would deliver sedatives. Usually I staved off my nerves by chatting with them. I'd joke about my fear of needles, lightly question the skills of my surgeons or ask how they got into nursing, but instead I lay there silently watching them perform their tasks. The valium in my IV bag sent me drifting off to sleep before I even realized I was sleepy and I didn't wake up until the next day. I woke disoriented and in more pain than I had ever imagined but was grateful for the excellent hospital staff dispensing regular doses of pain medication, attempting to ease my distress.

My mom was there and the minute my eyes opened, she said, "I had a dream the night before your surgery. You were being chased by a bear that Simon and Abner were fighting off. The bear finally ran away."

My mom hardly ever dreamt, but when she did she usually found some sort of message. Her interpretation of her new dream was that my cancer was gone, but silently I thought "gone for now."

Later that day, one of the nurses came to report that according to the insurance company I was ready to be released. However, it was the opinion of the nursing team, that it just wasn't possible for me to go home. They were trying to make it so I could stay but didn't know how since there was no primary doctor listed for my discharge. It had become a point of confusion because I had so many doctors working on me at different times, performing different primary surgeries.

"You'll figure it out," I said with a weak smile. "Because you won't be able to get me out of this bed."

The nurse and I laughed together, and I really did have faith they'd sort it out. I began to take stock of all that my body had just endured then fell asleep. I woke up at the shift change and a new nurse came in with my discharge papers. She must've recognized the alarmed look on my face and started to explain that the insurance company wanted me out that day, adding that it was very normal.

I said, "I know, but I'm supposed to stay until tomorrow. You need to find my doctor."

It was mind blowing that the insurance company I had faithfully paid premiums to month after month could quibble over pennies. I wondered if it was made clear to them that I had just suffered three surgeries in one. I had two rubber grenade-like drains full of body fluid hanging off my gown tethered by stretchy tubes that disappeared into my skin just under where my breast had been. My pain level on a scale from 0-10 was at "excruciating," and I couldn't possibly move. I pleaded with the nurses to find Dr. Doering right away.

Within the hour, the nurse returned to my room with a message that Dr. Doering had refused to discharge me. On his orders, a call was made to the insurance company and an extra day of hospital recovery time was secured. I was so grateful. The news that I'd be cared for one more day took the edge off my pain or maybe the accumulation of pain medicine added to my IV was finally working. Either way, I drifted off to sleep without a care in the world.

In the early evening, I woke to the nurses outside my door discussing my follow-up care. Once again, there was confusion over who my lead doctor would be. Dr. Doering had deferred to Dr. Sanders, Dr. Sanders deferred back to Dr. Doering and I decided to stop listening. I left it to them to work it out because it didn't matter to me one way or the other. Just then, my primary nurse Tammy showed up in such a cheery mood and made me laugh at what she called the "whole ABBOT and COSTELLO routine" playing out in the hall.

"Who's on first. What's on second. Who's on first?" she said giggling.

It hurt to laugh, causing me to feel dizzy and nauseous again, so she quickly tucked me in and ordered me to sleep with a wink and a smile.

April 7, 2006
In the afternoon of the second day after surgery, I was given thorough instructions on how to keep the drains clean and which activities I was not allowed to perform before being wheeled out to the waiting car where Ron helped me into the front seat and carefully drove me home. Every single bump in the road or turn of the corner was unbearable even on the concoction of pain medication coursing through my veins. Periodically, I realized I was gripping the door so tightly that I had to consciously let out a breath to release it, then I'd doze until the next bump or turn jerked me awake. At home, my mom was waiting to help me up the stairs to my bedroom. When I walked through the door, I was speechless. My room was filled with a beautifully fragrant collection of flowers that immediately masked the smell of hospital permeating

out of my every pore.

Home sweet home.

I collapsed into our bed modified by Ron with blankets under the mattress that propped me up so I could sleep comfortably instead of trying to sleep in a recliner. He's like MacGyver sometimes with his ability to retrofit anything to meet our needs.

Suzannah called and seemed to need to say, "Isn't it strange how our relationship has evolved? I can't really remember a time when you weren't around."

That warmed my heart. There's a 13-year age gap between us, and an unexpected silver lining from cancer was that it gave us an opportunity to grow closer. She was truly a special and amazing gift to me. With all of the love and support around me, I couldn't help but feel better. My arm and chest were still very sore, but it didn't seem to matter as much.

Ron slept in the guest room not wanting to bump me in his sleep since he could be a thrasher during a dream and had been known to clock me in the head or face. On the other hand, I would've liked him there for comfort. If I needed anything, he'd be right there, but in the end, the pain medication kept me subdued and before long it was morning and Ron was at the door checking in.

As I began to come to life I noticed that EmmaGrace was having a harder time. It was like she was disappointed that I appeared weak. Even though I begged her to come into my room and say hello, she wouldn't, leaving Ron to intervene by explaining to her that I'd heal a lot faster with lots of love. So ever the thespian, EmmaGrace threw herself into the role.

"HI, MOMMY! HOW ARE YOU? CAN I GET YOU ANYTHING?" She said over enunciating very loudly.

"No, I'm fine. I'm just happy to see your smiling face. I love you soooo much," I responded from the bed, trying to match her energy.

I held out my hand hoping she would take it but instead she yelled, "Ok. LOVE YOU TOO!" and ran out of the room.

If I was sitting downstairs and EmmaGrace noticed me looking at her, she would plaster a quick smile on her face. Then she would sing, "I love you, Mommy!" and run off before I could engage her in any meaningful way. I kept myself covered with blankets to hide the scars and drains, but their weight was terribly uncomfortable. On the other hand, it seemed necessary to shield her from my transformation into the "Bride of Frankenstein." Relief came only when she left the room and I could throw off the blankets and let out a big breath before collapsing into the mattress. I wanted to make everything OK and give her a big hug, but the fear of pain was overwhelming. She must've felt somewhat abandoned because before cancer came to town she loved to snuggle with me while I stroked her head and forehead. I loved to be close to her, but in an instant it all had changed, and I could only imagine how confusing that must've been for her.

Ron was my caretaker. He cleaned the drains, recorded the amount of fluid on the log sheet and washed out the clotted, gelatinous blood gunk from the top of the grenade before reattaching the whole contraption. He pinned the grenades back to my shirt and left me to fall back to sleep assisted by the emotional exhaustion of it all. I couldn't imagine how he would ever look at me the same way, but I never said those words out loud. I did draw the line at washing myself. I wouldn't let him help me with that. Instead, I waited until the house was empty before making my way to the shower. I had to keep the incisions dry, so I wet a rag and tenderly washed my skin around the bandages, resisting the urge to rip them off and wash the itchy skin healing underneath. The entire process took me nearly an hour and left me exhausted once again.

April 10, 2006.
I found myself back in Dr. Sanders's office, to have the bandages removed.

Without even looking at my face he said, "Everything looks great. It's healing very nicely."

He was almost talking out loud to himself, praising his own work. In response, I gave a weak smile that he never even saw. Dr. Sanders applied new bandages and set a schedule to begin filling the expander with saline, explaining that each subsequent visit would involve adding more of the salt solution, which would cause my skin to stretch. When "we" had reached the target size, he would insert a permanent implant.

"Target size?" I questioned.

"Yes, you're a D or DD right now, so we'll get the other side there as well," he stated as if it was a done deal and never asking what I wanted.

"Can I not go that big?" I asked.

"Well, I suppose. But then you'll need to have a reduction on the left side to get them as close as possible," he answered with less conviction.

Admittedly, I had no idea what any of that meant and I didn't care. I just wanted to go home and climb into bed, which was my well-worn mode of avoidance. I stopped asking questions and began to stand up. Dr. Sanders instructed me that the next day I was to remove the bandages over the holes where the grenades were and then he took his leave.

April 11, 2006
Everyone was out for the day and I made my way to the bathroom to remove the final bandages. I stood in front of the mirror staring at my face, working to not look down at my chest. Ron said he couldn't care less about what I looked like and while I appreciated his support, I wasn't sure I believed him let alone believed myself when I said the same. At one point during my treatment, I had joined an online chat group for breast cancer patients. I had only read through some of the past posts when I hit a wall. One of the discussions going on was about women whose husbands cheated on them during their battle or left their wives all together. It was completely beyond my comprehension how someone could be so heartless. I closed out that site and never returned, but the possibility of Ron leaving stuck like the barb of a burr in my brain.

I took my sponge bath and afterwards stood in front of the mirror with the towel covering my wounds. "OK!" I yelled out loud. Then, I looked under my arm for any red line that might indicate an infection and out of nowhere I heard Helen Reddy singing in my head. I spontaneously joined in at the top of my lungs.

"I am woman hear me roar in numbers too big to ignore, and I know too much to go back to pretend!"

I laughed so hard at myself and then sang the entire song as loudly as I could. I didn't even know I knew all the words, but I did.

I sang the refrain over and over, "I can do anything! I am strong. I am invincible! I am woman!"

Yes, I did pay the price, but look how much I had gained – Life! Empowered by Helen's song, I studied the lines of red scars as I stood in front of that same mirror the tumor had been revealed in. There were fewer scars than I had imagined, and the space where my breast had been looked like an eye winking back at me as if to say, "You've got this." I got dressed and still had enough energy to call for my pathology results from the surgically removed tissue.

I called Dr. Tousignant who jubilantly reported, "Your ovaries are clean as a whistle!"

Next, I called Mary at the cancer center who read part of my report over the phone but needed Dr. Harper to call me later because there was confusion with the results. I felt slightly deflated but hung up just in time to answer Dr. Doering's call.

"The breast tissue was clean," he reported.

He no longer said "your breast." It had been turned over to the lab and belonged to them. It wasn't anonymous just not part of a human being. It felt odd to divest myself of my breast. It felt even more strange to think of it being sliced, diced and studied closely under a microscope without my body anywhere in the vicinity.

"But 3 of 8 nodes were involved." Dr. Doering continued.

In other words, they still had cancer in them. Suddenly I went into a feeding frenzy of questions.

"How could the cancer have survived the chemo?" I asked over and over.

"If it was in the nodes, could the cancer cells have escaped to other parts of my body?"

Dr. Doering answered by saying he had no good answers for me at that moment but suggested I may have to have more chemotherapy because there was cancer that had metastasized outside of the nodes as well. I almost hung up without even saying good-bye as my mind raced. I had believed that surgery was the final hurrah. The big shebang. The grand finale. Now what? The cancer was in my dermis or skin, but by sheer luck it hadn't crossed paths with any of my dermal lymphatics. In 2005, my report classified me as stage IV, but I recently learned that the staging has changed in the last 10 years and in 2015 they might've staged me at IIIC with a survival rate of just over four years since the definition of metastases had changed. Today, the only qualified metastases are in the lungs, brain, liver or bones, but as with everything in the cancer world, staging was also fluid. Cancer research was an ever-evolving field and I was grateful every day for the scientists dedicating their talents to ending it once and for all. Unfortunately for me at the time, we were operating with a stage IV diagnosis and I spun out of control into another anxiety attack.

I was so scared and my earlier words came back to me. "If this cancer survives after everything we've thrown at it, then I guess it wins."

I yelled at myself and up to the universe, "What a stupid thing to say. I take it back! I'm not going to quit. I'm not a loser. I'm not a quitter. I take it all back! I swear I'm in it to win it!!"

I repeated those last six words over and over out loud. The phrase became my new mantra and I found myself saying it every waking hour. "I'm in it to win

it! Do you hear me?"

April 12, 2006
A week after my surgery, there was so much confusion, and Suzannah wanted answers that the pathologist hadn't given.

The report read, "Three out of eight lymph nodes are positive for metastatic carcinoma (3/8); two of the positive nodes show extra-nodal extension; largest metastatic focus measures 1.0 cm."

Suzannah wanted to know which level of nodes had cancer present. Was it in the sentinel nodes, my lymph system's first line of defense and closest to the cancer, or had the cancer gained deeper access? Dr. Harper explained to me that the nodes had become a sort of sanctuary for the cancer, which had blocked the blood flow and therefore chemo from entering. Although, no one was 100% clear on the location of the nodes to the tumor, the pathologist and surgeon felt they were most definitely sentinel nodes and the cancer hadn't made it to any others. While that offered Suzannah some amount of relief, I focused my attention on the rogue cells that may have slipped through the front lines to infiltrate the rest of my body.

April 20, 2006
As time marched on, I no longer needed the Zofran for nausea, which meant I had a pile of it left. It was such an expensive drug and it seemed like a complete waste to throw it away. When I was first prescribed the medication, the insurance company limited how many they would give me. To get more I had to fill out a special application explaining my need. I mean why would an insurance company want to make anything easy for a cancer patient? So, between Mary and Ron spending a combined 15 hours on the phone with them, arguing over my need to take several each day, the company agreed to send me 80 pills but no more. When their package arrived a day or two later, it was filled with 250 pills. I couldn't believe their stupidity. After all of their whining about cost, they had sent me more than four times what I had requested and only charged me for 80. I admit, however, I did relish that moment a little bit.

When I had used all of the Zofran that I could, I offered it to the cancer clinic for people who weren't able to get it through their insurance company. Yes, that's right. Some people weren't allowed to have it because it was too expensive. Unfortunately while they would've liked to, federal law precluded doctors from taking extra pills from patients if they were not individually wrapped. That left me to forge an agreement with my team that they were welcome to give my phone number to anyone who wanted the pills and I would personally deliver them. I was thrilled that Dr. Tousignant was the first to take me up on it.

"Do you still have the extra Zofran?" she asked over the phone.

"I do. I have more than I could ever take." I eagerly responded.

"Well, I have a patient with a couple of small children. She is pregnant with her third and suffering terrible nausea. She's been hospitalized multiple times because her insurance company won't pay for Zofran," she sputtered with disgust.

"So, it's better if she has to have somebody take care of her kids while she lays in a hospital bed receiving fluids? Isn't that a lot more expensive?" I asked.

"Of course it is. It's stupid. Could I give her your number?" she asked somewhat rhetorically.

"Absolutely! I would be happy to send her some," I agreed and hung up the phone.

Helping someone else made me feel good and gave me a big boost of energy. I got the woman's address and Ron sent the Zofran out right away. I never heard how she did, but I trusted she didn't have any more hospital stays before her baby was born.

Easter 2006
My parents brought dinner over on Easter elevating my spirit with the celebratory atmosphere. After dinner, Ron took the girls for a walk outside so my parents and I could chat without interruption. They were so devoted to their children and grandchildren, and I loved them deeply for it. Tears welled up in their eyes as they told me how much they wished they could do more for me. I couldn't begin to imagine what they were going through, and I felt so sad for them. I assured them they were already doing so much for us and thanked them for everything but decided the only way I could truly thank them was to live.

113

So, I once again promised I would be fine.

At bedtime, EmmaGrace cried. I was so physically and emotionally exhausted by then that I was afraid to ask what was wrong. Thankfully, the mother in me had to.

"Peanut, why are you upset?" I gently asked.

"I'm mad at you," she responded looking down.

"Why are you mad at me," I asked hoping to offer her comfort in my willingness to let her speak.

"I'm having terrible dreams. In them I'm hitting you so hard that you die. Well, I'm not really sure if I killed you or you died of something else," she answered as her shoulders relaxed.

Admittedly a little horrified by what I had heard, I squashed my own feelings down and told her I understood how scared she must be and how angry she must feel.

"I'm mad at you! I'm mad at God! I hate the kids at school!" she proclaimed through her tears.

Then, she launched into a story about how mean her classmates had become. I just couldn't resist and held her, trying to be mindful of the love and block out the pain in my chest. I felt incapacitated as a mother. I knew I wasn't really there for her the way she needed me, but I tried.

April 26 2006
About three weeks after surgery, I had both drains removed and braced for the first tissue expansion. I never could have anticipated how much it was going to hurt while Dr. Sanders injected the saline. I noticed a slight smile trying to push its way onto his face. Much like a parent might smile when their child screams in pain at the quick removal of a Band Aid. He of course would never know the true pain of the expansion process, but having seen so many women go through it, he knew I'd survive.

Later that day, Ron broke his ankle as I wallowed in pain from the expansion, and EmmaGrace cried herself to sleep. That was life in our home over run with cancer. It never seemed to end. A couple days later, EmmaGrace contracted the stomach flu, and a huge seroma filled with bloody fluid developed at my mastectomy site. While it wasn't necessarily dangerous it did provide an additional layer of discomfort, leaving me vulnerable to slip back into despair and left to wonder if all those little nit-picky events would break us. Then just in the nick of time, Hannah danced into view, flashing her loving smile, twirling and singing until I couldn't help but smile back.

Hannah's technique to bring happiness into our home gave me one of my better ideas during that time. I thought of a new way to "play" with my girls. Since we all loved music, I turned on an upbeat channel and invited them into the living room for a "dance party." Standing on the floor next to them, I waved my good arm around shuffling my feet back and forth while they bounced and twirled around me screeching with joy. I stood like that as long as possible and then collapsed into a chair clapping with the music. The smile on my face was real. There was no faking the way they made me feel as they administered the best medicine I could have ever had.

Ron took the dance party as a sign that we were getting back to some sort of normal and decided to host another rocket party with his brothers. We had started those parties 13 years before at our first house in Oconomowoc, WI, and had taken a couple of years off because of my compromised health. They were always in the dead of winter with the purpose of brightening up the doldrums, and it was always such a festive day punctuated by a chili dump and prizes given for the "The Most Creative," "The Least Likely To Fly But Still Does," "The Best Explosion," and "The People's Choice" among others. The crowds had reached upwards of 250 people and the chaos was hysterical. I loved the event, and since we didn't allow anyone to come to the party without a rocket, it offered a great way to get parents doing something creative with their kids Ron's brothers promised I wouldn't have to lift a finger and remained true to their word. Before the crowd arrived, friends came to help set up and organize. No sooner was I expressing how happy I was to see them when my irrational paranoia struck. I was sure they were giving me the "it's all over look," but of course they weren't. Overwhelmed by my own insecurities, I retreated to my bedroom where I lay in bed listening as our house and yard flooded with enthusiastic rocketeers.

Once the launch began, the whooshing sound of rockets blasting into the air pulled me from my bed to the window where I watch like Boo Radley, taking in the joyful faces of laughing rocketeers and kids wearing big bright smiles covering every inch of the yard. When a rocket blasted off, the crowd stopped what they were doing and with mouths agape gazed at the lifting projectile, waiting for the parachute to pop out. Sometimes the rocket would explode or take a circuitous route on its flight, but it was a sure bet every launch would be met with the same ooh's, aah's, raucous laughter and admiration. From the window I planned how I would sneak unnoticed and melt in among the revelers while the party was in full swing, and the beer was flowing.

I took a deep breath, left the isolation of my room and made my way downstairs, hoping everyone was outside, but they weren't. There were flowers everywhere scattered throughout the kitchen and family room just like at a funeral. I noticed a pile of gifts covering the table in the living room as if it was my birthday, and by the time I hit the last step, it was too late to turn back. The gift givers milling around and talking to my parents had spotted me. By then I was well rehearsed in the art of plastering a fake smile on and feigned graciousness as I made my way through the crowd acknowledging the kind gifts and wishes for a quick recovery.

The phrase "God only gives you what you can handle," surfaced often.

Each time I heard it, I smiled weakly and eventually broke through the back door and outside to study each of the hand-made rockets lined up along the edge of the deck ready to be judged. I laughed out loud at the Martha Stewart rocket painted in black and white stripes and completed with a disheveled blonde wig, looking much like the one I had worn. She was in jail at the time and an attorney friend was the proud creator. The variety of rockets in all different shapes and sizes reminded me more of an adult science fair than a party. Even though the kids were involved in the construction, inevitably the dads had taken over.

I endured a couple of awkward high energy hours inundated with merriment before retiring back to my room, leaving EmmaGrace to take over as hostess. It was a role she relished. I quickly fell asleep, trying not to think about the incredible mess I would find when I awoke. It was a mess I had cleaned well into the wee hours of the morning for many years. However, when I tentatively made my way downstairs in the morning, nothing was out of place. I was dumbfounded until Ron appeared and said his brother's cleaning lady had taken care of it all.

"Why hadn't we ever done that before?" I asked laughing through my relief coupled with disbelief.

We spent the day making further adjustments to our living arrangements, so our lives would be more comfortable. Ron set to work on a new playroom for the girls in the basement, painting the walls a bright yellow and moving most of the toys into the cheery space where they could play loudly like children do. Upstairs, I sat in a chair, turned the music on and embraced my happy mood.

116

The girls heard the music and appeared in the living room with EmmaGrace declaring, "It's a dance party, Mommy!"

They were so happy, and I was infected by their joy. I ignored my fatigue and lifted my energy to meet theirs for just a minute before collapsing back onto the couch. It didn't matter to them how long I danced, just that I had.

Back to March 2006
On one sunny and relatively warm day in March, my neighbor Janet came over to sit with me on the deck. I welcomed the fresh air and her company equally. She didn't tiptoe around me like most visitors, trying to stay cheery as if making my final days more pleasant. They clearly could read the statistics on line just as easily as I could, and their inner dialogue must have been something like, "Her life expectancy is less than two years. Just keep it positive." Not Janet. She was in her own fight for life, and on that day, she began to share the traumatic stories of her marriage to a deranged and abusive man.

As long as I had known Janet I always had the feeling she was hiding something but had no clue that her secret would be as harrowing as it was. We were sitting on the deck warmed by the early spring sun and rocking in wooden chairs when she finally got real.

Thanks to cancer treatment I no longer had a filter and without any real sense of decorum and just blurted out, "Janet, are you living in an abusive marriage?"

She seemed shocked and terribly offended that I had said such a thing out loud. She fell silent, sitting quietly as she stared out over our south prairie.

When she finally spoke she looked right into my eyes and said, "Yes."

I told her why I had asked and that I had recognized some of what she was saying from the dialogue I had heard on television. With my many days spent on the couch I had just seen the Julia Roberts movie "Sleeping With The Enemy" along with way too many episodes of Dr. Phil exposing abusive husbands. I had always felt uneasy around Janet's husband Leonard and was about to learn why. My question broke the dam and Janet spilled the beans all over the place. She carefully described details about actions and conversations that had occurred during her life as a victim of spousal abuse. It was horrific. Leonard was maybe 21 years old when he began grooming Janet who was at the tender and impressionable age of 13. She lived in a chaotic household where her mother took care of the neighbor kids along with her own large brood, and Janet's alcoholic father grew marijuana in the basement of their family home. Showing incredible resilience, Janet hid out in her bedroom

117

reading or spending time at the library in an effort to just stay out of the fray. Leonard, a friend of her older brother, came to the house fairly often, and on one such occasion, he noticed Janet and immediately took a strong interest in her. Before long, he was hanging out with her regularly, and because Janet's parents were unable to see the warning signs, they settled into the comfort of knowing that someone was watching out for their sweet and reserved daughter.

As time went on, Leonard became more possessive over Janet, keeping her from social events with her friends. When she went to college he followed. It was there that he really dug in, keeping her from spending time with her family in any meaningful way. She was "not allowed" to be with friends unless he approved or was present. On some level I imagined Janet thought it was normal. After all, her parents seemed to like the "groomer" who she ended up marrying, naively committing herself to a life of abuse. Janet studied botany and horticulture while Leonard developed his career as a photographer. It wasn't long before he put his own work aside and directed her into developing a career in photography as well. As her pictures of wild and cultivated flora grew in popularity, Leonard controlled every aspect of her life. From the outside it looked like the perfect union. She was able to focus on her art while he handled the business. Unfortunately, the truth was not easily revealed to the few friends they socialized with because Janet had become masterful at covering up the physical, mental and emotional marks he left on her. I'm not sure that she ever believed she "deserved" it, but she stayed because she didn't see any way out. Janet was estranged from friends and family with Leonard serving as her stifling conduit to the world.

As soon as Leonard succeeded at isolating Janet, he locked up all of her personal records, including her birth certificate, health records, and bank statements. He had a car key made with the stamp "DO NOT DUPLICATE" only giving it to her with her driver's license, if he approved of where she was going. His cruelty became severe relatively quickly. His irrational anger sent Janet to sleep on the hard wood floor without a blanket or pillow. He harmed her physically over and over and subjected her to life threatening situations with some level of regularity because, as he repeated his mantra, "you deserve this punishment." Meanwhile, his paranoia that she might run grew, and he began to sleep in his jeans with the car keys tucked deep in his front pocket. Janet suffered in silence for 30 years and somehow managed to produce award-winning art in the process. She ran away a few times, and each time he hunted her down by charming her acquaintances into telling him where she was and then punishing her severely. As I listened to her shed the details of her imprisonment, my protective nature took hold. I felt stronger than I had in a long time and told her I would get her out. Her face showed utter disbelief and then fear. She wasn't afraid for herself, she was afraid for me.

118

"Janet, I have no fear of him. He's a bully with control only because you give it to him. Like all bullies, once you expose them they shrink back into the shadows," I said lovingly.

In the weeks to follow, we plotted what we would do. Janet was afraid to file charges against Leonard, believing the police would not take action to protect her, so periodically, she packed a bag of her things and left them at my house or with other people she knew on the days he allowed her to leave the house alone. During that time, Leonard seemed to know something was a foot but never suspected me as an accomplice. Using fear to keep her home, he threatened to burn the negatives from her life's work. When she told me, I went out to the store and purchased oversized Ziplock bags to hold her cherished negatives and kept them safely tucked away at my house guarded by our Irish wolfhound Skip. Because of my weakened state, I was the only one Leonard allowed Janet to visit. I called her often, feigning my need for help with the girls. He assumed I wouldn't have the energy to aid Janet in any way, but his psychotic ego couldn't have been further off the mark. I recalled my middle school social studies teacher writing on the board one day in very big letters, "ASS U ME."

He waited for us to all stop giggling and then said, "When you ASSUME, you make an ASS out of U and ME."

That was Leonard. In his case, however, he was the only ASS. Janet's needs energized me and became a powerful distraction from my daily life which would otherwise have been mired in self-pity. One day when Leonard went to the hardware store, Janet called me to say we had about 45 minutes before he'd be back, so I rushed over to her house and went to work in the basement, searching for her personal records. She led me to a line of file cabinets on the north wall, and one that was locked drew my attention for obvious reasons.

"I want to look in there," I said.

"I don't know where the key is," Janet replied helplessly.

"No need. I had this type of file cabinet in my office. I can get in," I assured her.

Grateful for what I called my chemo pants, maroon, stretchy, elastic waist band pants, I pressed my foot to the front outside edge of the cabinet and gripped the drawer handle as tightly as I could. Janet stood behind me offering support in case I lost my balance, and with a deep breath I focused all of my strength on pulling back with a hard jerk. The drawer lock popped, leaving its contents open for us to dive into. There were bank statements Janet had never seen. She had no idea how much money she had and was shocked to see the numbers. Let's just say Janet was going to be quite financially comfortable once we got her out of there. Leonard had never let her buy anything new always forcing her to buy clothes, furniture and other household items at second hand shops.

We wrote down the banks and account numbers then identified her health records, which we could make copies of on another day. We took copies of some news articles announcing her awards in photography to present at the banks as proof of identity since her birth certificate was nowhere to be found. He had probably burned it in the bonfire he constantly tended out behind the barn. Once we knew what was in those drawers, we closed them back up and I scurried home to make some calls. One of my friends had recently told me that she wanted to buy one of Janet's photographs but had such a hard time picking one out amongst the art show crowds where Leonard had them displayed. Remembering that she had asked if I thought they would let her go to their house to look at them, she was my first call. I explained Janet's situation and asked if she would call Leonard and ask if Janet could show them at my house. It was a perfect way to get her inventory out of the house without Leonard in tow. My friend called him right after we hung up and organized the date and time. Leonard instructed Janet to call me to organize the "showing," and I could hardly contain my excitement.

The next call was to a mutual friend of ours who worked in the financial world. He and his wife agreed to help Janet escape and had a place for her to safely stay. Terrified, Janet tried to delay the jailbreak, but Ron laid it on the line for her one night while she was "helping" me with the girls.

"Janet, you either have to shit or get off the pot, and I suggest you get off," he sternly counseled.

It was enough of a push to move Janet towards her day of liberation. I was really excited for her as I closely watched the clock. She was supposed to be at my house by 9:00 a.m. that day, but by 9:15 a.m., she still hadn't arrived. I paced between the front door and back window, watching for her van before deciding something was wrong. If Leonard had driven by and seen that my friend's car wasn't parked in the driveway, he would stop her from coming. I called their house and Janet answered. Deciphering her cryptic language, I surmised that Leonard had sensed something was awry but still did not suspect that I had anything to do with it. What had happened was that Janet lost her courage on the way out and walked to her car instead of the van containing her inventory. That was the red flag Leonard was watching for. Ironically, he told her she would not be taking her car because he was going to search it while she was at my house. Ultimately, he put her in the van full of inventory and off she drove. In the end, Leonard had aided Janet in her final escape. She arrived at my house shaking, hyperventilating and crying. I held her for a few minutes, asking her to try and synch her breathing with mine. We took slow and steady breaths in and slowly blew them out until she regained control of her body.

"Are you OK to drive?" I asked her.

"I'm not sure," she whispered.

"Well, you're going to have to be because Deb and Dan are waiting for you. I'll pull out of the driveway right behind you in case Leonard shows up and tries to stop you. YOU don't look back. Just drive and I'll block him from following," I ordered. "Now, let's go before we lose too much more time."

Janet drove out of my driveway and I followed closely behind, studying my rear view mirror constantly, but Leonard never appeared. I imagined him tearing through her car, digging like the dog he was down the wrong rabbit hole. He was trapped in a pattern he had created, but Janet had broken free. When I handed her off with Deb and Dan, they removed the license plates from her van and hid it in an outbuilding on their land. They immediately ushered her into their car and drove her to each of the banks holding her money. Unfortunately, times had changed and the banks no longer accepted newspaper articles as proof of identity, so the pair drove her to Milwaukee to get her birth certificate where they were thwarted once again because she needed some form of identification for that as well. The state said they would accept a marriage license, which Janet also did not have. So, off to Madison they drove where she managed to obtain a copy of her marriage license using her signature as proof of identity. Then, it was on to the Department of Motor Vehicles for a new driver's license. It was a bureaucratic rats nest working against the victim, and by the time she had her license in hand, the banks were closed. They would have to wait until the next morning to withdraw her money, and we knew Leonard knew she was gone. He never called me to ask if she had arrived because it would've most certainly exposed him. Dan knew Leonard couldn't freeze their accounts since it was a Friday night and he really had no reason to. The previous times Janet had "run away," she never withdrew money.

The next day, Dan and Deb took Janet back to her banks where she generously withdrew only half of the cash, reasoning that it was all the state would give her in a divorce anyway. We tried to explain she wasn't divorced and she could take more, but her fear was strong and wouldn't allow her to do that. With cash in hand, she purchased a car and moved into a safe house next to another woman who had also escaped from her abusive husband. While Dan and Deb organized Janet's finances, I organized her new home. I bought her some groceries and put them in the refrigerator, laid out some magazines I thought she might enjoy, put basil in a vase, some lavender bath salts in the bathroom, and a large lavender plant on the coffee table. Next to it I displayed some drawings the girls had made for her along with a photograph I took of them with Janet. I wanted her to feel our love, hoping it would be enough to keep her from going back to that vicious bully.

Saturday night, we all reconvened and went out for a celebratory dinner. The girls were a little confused by the whole ordeal that played out better than any movie I had ever seen. Janet was stunned by her network of support, realizing that all she had ever needed to do was make her cry for help. As soon as she voiced her intentions, her rescue boat quickly materialized with the strength of a massive earthquake rocking her world while destroying a part of Leonard's forever. For me, helping her took me from the weakness of cancer into a world where I still had purpose, and with one more awkward task ahead of me, I formulated how I was going to explain to the girls what had happened. I didn't want them to open the door if Leonard showed up at our house.

"EmmaGrace, if Leonard comes to the door I want you to run to me and we'll call 911. Don't talk with him, don't listen to what he has to say, just run." I emphatically insisted.

"What's wrong with Leonard?" she asked.

"Everything. No matter how well we think we know someone, a time can come when you realize you never knew them at all. Leonard has hurt Janet very badly and has threatened to kill her. He is a very dangerous person. He's also very sick. He threatened to suffocate Janet and then kill himself," I answered, wondering if I had told my eight-year-old too much.

EmmaGrace made a comment about how bad that was especially since Janet was such a nice person. Then, she walked away to find Hannah and play. Had I done the right thing? I didn't know, but I wouldn't have been able to live with myself had he come over and she let him in thinking he was still a friend. I've decided not to include more of Janet's sordid details here in hopes that one day she will tell her own story. I was so proud of what I was able to do for her and what she did for herself, and I would do it again in a heartbeat because she deserved nothing more than love and happiness. I never told her that she had given me a gift as well. Helping her take control of her life was like a jumpstart back into my own. Her challenge gave me a mission outside of myself, allowing me to see I still had worth.

Back to May 2, 2006

As always, I couldn't have the ups without the downs and another tissue expansion loomed around the corner. The healing of my wound had slowed way down, leaving the incision site partially open due to a lack of blood supply in my skin. Noticeably frustrated with me, Dr. Sanders explained that the scar would no longer be smallish, as if it was somehow my fault. I let his attitude roll off my back, but his next comment didn't slide so easily.

"There's no way you can start radiation on time with the wound still opened. Don't get me wrong. That's a good thing because it gives me more time to stretch your skin," Dr. Sanders stated as if my opinion carried no weight.

I didn't want to stretch my skin much more. The fact that every week I missed radiation was a week the cancer could grow unencumbered was enough nevermind the pain of tissue expansion. I decided to stop at B sized breasts. Bolstering my point of view was Dr. Harper who strongly believed that if I was going to stay ahead of the cancer, I had to start radiation soon. In the midst of disagreeing doctors, I couldn't help but remember the words of caution from Dr. Doering before my surgery.

"I understand you want to get on with the rest of your treatment, but putting the expander in before radiation isn't a great option. There are all kinds of complications that can arise, least of which is that the breast tissue can harden around the expander. I'd like you to consider waiting until after your radiation treatments," he counselled.

Desperate to finish my treatment, I ignored Dr. Doering's wise warning. Had I listened I might have been spared the mounting complications that were to arise. Being a cancer patient was incredibly difficult and confusing especially when there were so many conflicting opinions on my team. Initially, I naively thought of cancer treatment as a relatively straightforward process.

Unfortunately, it was anything but. If only there really was a "one size fits all" in the medical protocol box for cancer treatment, but there never would be. Everyone had their own cancer experience because every BODY was different. The more I engaged in pessimism, the harder my days became, which left me only one choice - shake off the desperation creeping in like a spider moving up my arm. I shuddered, said a prayer for strength, picked myself up by my invisible boot straps, and moved one more emotional step forward.

May 16, 2006

After more than a month, the incision site still hadn't healed, and with every stretch of the tissue expander the wound opened a little more. Janet bought a

123

herbal healing balm with calendula and comfrey at the People's Pharmacy in Madison, hoping it would do the job, but it didn't. At my next appointment, Dr. Sanders brought up the topic of breast size again. He was not at all concerned that each time he reached for size D, the incision broke open a little more, delaying the necessary radiation that I hoped would ensure my recovery.

"You realize the longer we delay my radiation treatments, the better the chances are that the cancer recurs? I can't afford that. I want to stop the expansion when it reaches a B," I said looking him straight in the eyes, reminding him that it was about me and my ultimate goal not his.

"I do," was all Dr. Sanders said in response.

I continued my regular appointments with Dr. Harper who asserted that he had a "good feeling" about my prognosis as long as I could get my radiation going. He set out a plan to do a follow-up mammogram and chest x-ray in November, which would clear the way for my last reconstructive surgery soon after. My forward mantra must've been rubbing off on him as well since he rarely looked that far out into the future. The original plan was for me to be done with radiation by July, but everything had been thrown up in the air because of the gaping wound where my cancer riddled breast had once been. My mental strength waivered with each passing day of delays, and the fear of recurrence constantly knocked at my door. I couldn't help but remember the lymph nodes clogged with cancer, the cells that had slipped outside of the nodes, and the likelihood that rogue cells were dividing somewhere in my body once again. I wanted a break from doctors, procedures, tests and surgeries before the one-year anniversary of my diagnosis, but that clearly wasn't going to happen. As I felt myself spiral back down into the pit of depression, I tossed a metaphoric grappling hook on the ledge and adjusted my attitude once again. The more prayer and meditation I did, the easier it became to right my ship.

Summer was in the air and seemingly joyful at the prospect of no more school, Hannah gave me random hugs throughout the day while EmmaGrace shared the occasional hug, causing my strength to coalesce once again. My hair wasn't growing as quickly as I would've liked, but I had come to enjoy the simplicity of it. I began to experiment with supplements instead of medications in an attempt to hold some control over cancer recurrence by adding cod liver oil, vitamin D3 and fish oil to my morning routine. I paid better attention to removing all processed sugar from my diet and tried to exercise a little bit every day. Living more mindfully allowed me to take notice of how I craved certain foods for a while before the craving would pass. For example, leading up to my diagnosis, I craved cranberry juice, but seven months into treatment, it never even crossed my mind. More recent studies have shown that cranberries carry the ability to kill cancer cells in the lab, and I wondered if it had done the same for me in the wild landscape of my infirm body. I began to listen closely to any and all hankerings, checking them against the list of cancer fighting foods posted in my kitchen. More often than not, the food was listed. I knew it sounded a little crazy to most people in my life, but I was certain that learning to listen very closely to my body was feeding my recovery.

In our small backyard garden, I played around with the list of anti-angiogenic foods, curious to see how hard it would be to grow and harvest them ourselves. In a short time, I realized the garden wasn't big enough to feed our family of four, so we joined a CSA in the neighboring town to supplement our supply. A local farmer had set up a program formally called Community Supported Agriculture or CSA, in which we were allowed to purchase a subscription to his farm in exchange for fresh produce each week throughout the growing season. The first crop was asparagus and it tasted like nothing I had ever had before. I mean, I had eaten asparagus before but none that tasted like his. Each vegetable or fruit we found in our bag had the same effect. The flavors were deeper and more satisfying than their grocery store counterparts simply because of the way they were grown.

The weekly trips to our CSA became a coveted family outing during which we'd stroll along the bark-covered paths through his organized raised beds of colorful produce. We dodged chickens as they scurried out from under our feet and sampled vegetables that we picked right from the plant. I found a profound joy in the way the girls gobbled up vegetables they had never eaten before. Cherry tomatoes and spinach leaves disappeared into their mouths like

candy as their little hands worked faster and faster ` to pick as much as they could before we had to go home. It was clear none of us had tasted anything better...ever. As I learned more about how the food was grown, it began to make sense to me. Everything was organically grown and of an heirloom variety, meaning it hadn't been artificially genetically modified. No toxic pesticides or herbicides had been used on the plants or in the soil, which made a huge difference in the flavor and nutritional quality of their yield. That CSA opened our eyes to a whole new world of culinary delights and inspired me to cook fresh every day. Together, we enthusiastically pledged to expand our little home garden the following year and add chickens into the mix and intentionally became subsistence farmers.

May 19, 2006
Unfortunately, I wasn't allowed to bask too long in that blissful moment of freedom from the medical community before it came to an abrupt end with Dr. Harper prescribing the next drug that was assigned to "help" me heal. During

that appointment, he recapped the previous months by congratulating me for completing dose dense chemotherapy, enduring disfiguring and debilitating surgeries, and working hard to beat back any possibility of recurrence. He was also happy I had found a "distraction" in food, but he wanted me to stay the course and add the post-chemo drug called Tamoxifen.

"Since we know your estrogen and progesterone receptors were positive, we can have you start taking Tamoxifen. It's a drug widely used to block hormone receptors in breast cancer cells which inhibit the mechanism cancer uses to grow and divide. But unfortunately, Tamoxifen comes with substantial side effects that I need you to understand. They include an increased risk of uterine cancer and the development of blood clots, but I truly believe the benefits outweigh the risks," Dr. Harper said, pausing to give me a chance to respond.

"Do they really? I had my ovaries removed to avoid taking any more drugs. I mean, aren't I already free of hormones, having had my ovaries removed?" I asked.

"Well, why don't you start taking it, and I'll do some further research. Is that a deal?" he asked rhetorically.

Almost as soon as I started Tamoxifen, Dr. Harper took me off, replacing it with an aromatase inhibitor. There was so much information for him to weigh, and after looking further into my options, he realized that Tamoxifen was primarily designed for patients that had not gone into menopause like I had following my first chemotherapy dose back in December. In addition, I was down one pair of ovaries that would have otherwise been producing the majority of my body's hormones. However, Dr. Harper explained that my adrenal glands were still producing as much as 20% of the hormones my body used, and the aromatase inhibitors were designed to end that estrogen production, leaving the cancer completely starved of proteins.

Aromatase inhibitors also targeted the enzyme (aromatase) in fat cells, which produced small amounts of estrogen in post-menopausal women. Since I no longer had my ovaries, Dr. Harper agreed I could try a variety of drugs in that series including Arimidex, Femara and finally Aromasin. First up was Arimidex. It was terrible. The pain was so intense, I found it impossible to function in any productive way during the day. So, we threw it in the trash, and I took a short break to recover from its side effects before rebooting with Femara. Sadly, it produced the same horrendous pain which left Aromasin as my only option. While the resulting pain was no walk in the park, I was at least able to function. I had no choice but to grin and bear it for an undetermined number of years until something better came along. It was undeniably clear that

126

my body had developed a high sensitivity to prescription medications, which left me to manage a multitude of side-effects, including some that were considered rare, just like my cancer. While I was willing to tolerate the pain, increased nausea, extreme fatigue and dizziness brought to me courtesy of Aromasin, it was the "mood swings" as they were described on the manufacturer's fact sheet that were impossible to endure. In my case, the aforementioned mood swings looked more like intense rage.

Our home had become a war zone and relief came only when I removed myself completely to hide out in my bedroom, which was the only place I could slip away from my ugly reality. I halted my practice of meditation and mindfulness, choosing to replace it with self-pity and isolation in an effort to mitigate the impact of cancer on my family. It wasn't a good choice, but my judgment was clouded, so it seemed like my only choice.

May 25, 2006
It took six weeks before the expander incision had finally closed, except for one cavernous hole that provided an excellent view of my chest wall muscle. Clearly the hole showed no hope of healing and I begged my plastic surgeon to stitch it closed already so I could get on with the rest of my treatment. He reluctantly agreed, debrided the edges, stitched me up and handed the baton off to the radiation doctor. It was so easy that I wondered why he hadn't done it before. Threadbare from the ongoing onslaught of medical manhandling, I found myself in Radiation Oncologist Dr. Arnold's exam room. He was friendly and informative as he explained what he would do and what the potential recurrence rate was for cancer to return on the chest wall. My eyes drooped and no questions rose to my lips. I was too worn out to look in my notebook, turning the rest of his "orientation" to static. Dr. Arnold led me to the next exam room where the radiation technicians took measurements of my body to program their machine with my personal specifications before sending me on my way. The best I could do was smile weakly and thank them quietly as I trudged out the door. In hindsight, I probably should've listened more intently to Dr. Arnold because in the end, I suffered all of the side effects he had described - spontaneous rib fractures, lung damage and capsular contraction. Capsular contraction occurred when radiated tissue around the implant thickened, forming a capsule. In my case, the capsule not only formed but became like a suit of armor eventually distorting the shape of my reconstructed breast.

May 30, 2006
The weekend arrived like it always had, giving me something to count on without question, and I relished it like nothing else. During that time in my life, I was living a double life. Weekdays were given over to beating cancer and

weekends were given to my kids. The positive energy I exuded in the early part of my treatment was drained from my body, leaving me primarily quiet around my medical team so that when the weekend arrived, I could spill what little I had over my family. Ron worked to identify easy activities for us to do, including a canoe ride down the Rock River running just a couple miles from our house. The Saturday we paddled was a beautiful sunny day and the river swelled from the spring rains. The girls eagerly embraced their new paddling skills and joyously dipped their wooden paddles into the muddy river water, splashing each other as they pulled it them out. It was their first trip through that mystical watery sanctuary, flowing through the forests and farm fields so close to our home. Its banks hosted a variety of large birds including great blue herons, bitterns, sand hill cranes and bald eagles, nesting high above its shores. At times we pulled our paddles out of the water and speaking only in whispers let the current quietly carry us as we searched for fairies in the trees. Our boat's movement across the surface of the water caused the birds to startle from their perches before settling back down into our silence.

June 5, 2006

On another weekend, I found the strength to ride my bike along the Wild Goose Trail in Dodge County. It was part of the Wisconsin Rails to Trails system built over an abandoned rail road grade. Ron attached the tag-along bike to his for EmmaGrace, then the Burley trailer for Hannah behind that.

Hannah squealed with delight over EmmaGrace "pulling her," and EmmaGrace exclaimed, "Daddy made a bike train!"

All I had to do was peddle my own bike, managing to make it almost five miles before a terrible pain took hold in my right arm. My shirt sleeve became very tight and my arm was swollen and achy as if stung by a wasp. I hadn't felt a poke or any kind of pain from a bite, but surely something had bitten me.

"Can't I even just go for a bike ride with my family without something going wrong?" I bemoaned looking up to the clouds.

We back tracked to the car where Ron helped me search for the unprovoked sting until a light bulb went off in my head, and I realized it was lymphedema caused by the removal of my lymph nodes during the mastectomy. Even though I had been warned that it could come at any time after surgery, it had already been two months and I was sure I was out of the woods. Standing next to my bike, I was doused in another wave of vulnerability and cried.

"How many more complications do I have to endure? Haven't I been through enough?" I asked Ron rhetorically.

June 7, 2006

The next appointment with Dr. Sanders to remove the stitches, was wonderfully uplifting. Without a babysitter, EmmaGrace was forced to tag along. It was a good day for me because I loved her company, and while waiting to be called, I set her up in the waiting room with books and toys, introduced her to the friendly women at the receptionist's desk, and expected to leave her there thoroughly engaged throughout my appointment. However, when I was called in to the exam room, she popped up and glued herself to my side. I giggled with surprise, wrapped my arm around her soaking in the joy of having her there as my moral support, and completely forgot what she was about to witness while I basked in her affection. When Dr. Sanders arrived in the exam room, he was obviously surprised to see EmmaGrace and took a step back before proceeding in. He had kids of his own, so once he regrouped his demeanor, he skillfully navigated the conversation with her.

"I'm going to remove some stitches from your mom's skin. Are you all right with that?" he respectfully inquired.

She nodded yes and so he began to cut each stitch with EmmaGrace peering over his shoulder.

"Would you like to help me," Dr. Sanders asked giving me a wink.

I couldn't believe what I had heard but was even more surprised when EmmaGrace responded with an enthusiastic, "Yes!"

She took the tweezers and scissors from the surgeon's hands and began to pull up each stitch, snip it and tug it out, placing it on the tray held by my plastic surgeon and mimicking his moves exactly.

When they were all out, Dr. Sanders shook her hand and said, "You have a steady hand. Perhaps you'll be a surgeon someday."

EmmaGrace beamed with pride and so did I. When she was as small as two years old, she was mesmerized by the medical shows, and I marveled at her utter focus on the screen as she watched surgical procedures even the strongest of adults would shudder at.

I turned my attention back to myself and said with solid footing, "I want to move things forward, so when I've reached a B cup, I'm done with the expansion.

"I know it's painful, but you're going to have to have the left side reduced to

129

make them match otherwise you'll develop back pain from the uneven weight. I really think we should keep going. I don't think you're thinking this through rationally," he said in a somewhat insulting tone.

What Dr. Sanders didn't recognize was that they were my breasts, and I owned every bit of pain he delivered with each stretch of my skin. My only worry was battling an aggressive cancer, and I wanted to get the radiation show on the road, so a B cup would have to do.

June 11, 2006

Back at the farm we all spent some time in the barn visiting the horses and cleaning their stalls. Ron cleaned out the two unused stalls in preparation for a pair of calves he was bringing home by week's end. After reading a number of books like Michael Pollan's *OMNIVORES DILEMMA* and Barbra Kingsolver's *ANIMAL, VEGETABLE, MIRACLE,* we had decided to go all in and clean up our diet by growing as much of our own food as we could, including meat. Of course, beef was where Ron's heart was and mine was with the chickens. The meat from both would be packed with Omega-3 fatty acids just because they grazed on our chemical free pastures. Livestock typically raised on feedlots, eats food they were not designed to eat, which

causes the meat to become very high in Omega-6 fatty acids and very low in Omega-3. Omega-6 was the culprit behind increasing inflammation in our bodies and consequently increasing our risk of developing chronic disease. Omega-3's were the more favorable of the fatty acids, reducing inflammation to protect us against chronic illness. So livestock grown naturally, grazing on clean pasture, produced meat high in Omega-3 fatty acids, which would play a strong role in protecting us against a host of chronic diseases.

I continued my studies into the different theories on food as medicine, and after reading a number of different books including a series by Dr. Andrew Weil, I realized that reducing inflammation in my body was the key to getting healthy again. Inflammation was the precursor to disease and controlling it was something I absolutely would have to do if I was to prevent a cancer recurrence. We planned to expand our home garden the following spring into the outdoor arena where the girls and I had previously ridden our horses. Since, I wasn't really riding any more, its highly fertile soil would be ideal for growing produce packed with a disease-fighting punch. Ron bought a rototiller attachment for the tractor and plowed a total of 16 rows approximately 60 feet in length. Just like flipping through the old Sears Christmas catalogue when I was a child, I felt the warmth of the growing season upon us. I turned page after page in the organic seed catalogues, making a list of what I wanted to buy. As I cross referenced my selections with the anti-angiogenic food list developed with my research friends, our gardening list grew. I calculated the square footage of our garden, planning how much of each fruit or vegetable we could cultivate, then I mapped it out on paper, calculating our anticipated yield. When I was all done, it was clear we would have far more fresh produce than we could possibly eat, which meant we'd be learning how to can and freeze the rest for use during the winter months. The mere thought of becoming self-sufficient made me happier than I had been for almost an entire year. I recalled my secret ambition when we had bought that farm. I wanted to become as self-sufficient as possible, and it finally seemed like we were on our way.

To be expected, as soon as I allowed myself to feel joy, the cancer shoved past the happiness, hogging the scene. Suzannah called to tell me she had decided to take me to the University of Wisconsin-Madison for a second opinion on Aromasin and any further testing or treatments I might need. She spent hours organizing my medical records into the format preferred by research doctors by placing a red sheet of paper between each section, dividing the file into my tests, treatments, blood work and surgeries to date.

"I have complete faith in Dr. Harper. Why would I need to go to Madison?" I asked.

"He's reviewing everything through his filter. A fresh perspective might be a good idea," she replied with compassion.

It wasn't a tough choice for me since I had more faith in Suzannah than all of my doctors combined. She was looking at me as a person not a protocol. So if that was what she thought was best, then that was what I would do. We scheduled my appointment for the fall after I was done with the grueling radiation treatments. Since IBC had invaded my skin, I would have to endure having my skin completely burned off. I truly couldn't imagine what that would mean, but everyone said radiation was a breeze compared to chemo, so I chose to believe them.

June 14, 2006
I turned my attention to the other elephant in the room. The 25 pounds I had added to my frame began producing hormones that could be used by the cancer, which was entirely unacceptable to me. I began to watch my weight very carefully, trying to lose whatever I could and weighing myself at home in the privacy of my bathroom. It was a step up from the humiliating weigh-ins at the cancer center, which took place at each visit on the scale in the main hall. The first time I weighed myself, I gingerly stepped on the scale, anticipating a higher number than the week before. I drew in a breath, then slowly cast my eyes down to the digital screen where I struggled to comprehend what I was

131

reading. I had lost three whole pounds. While it wasn't 25 pounds, three pounds was three pounds.

I bounced out of the bathroom and twirled around chattering as I ran to tell Ron who was outside on the deck, "I'm getting better. I'm getting better!"

Each of those little positives became monumental in my life, and I searched for them everywhere. I found another one just outside my back door. On the deck, Ron heard the cry of an endangered black crowned night heron nesting in one of our pines trees.

"Listen. It calls in intervals," He said shushing me.

"I lost three pounds," I whispered back.

He gave me a thumbs up and then put his index finger to his lips. The heron called again. I squinted my eyes, searching the trees for the nest and marveled at the rarity of having a black crowned night heron fighting for existence on our farm. It was my distinct honor to provide a safe place for at least one pair. Although I couldn't actually see them, they felt like kindred spirits, which led me to another little positive moment. With Ron's help, I made a list of the wild animals sharing that little piece of land with us. Over the years, we had seen snowy owls, bald eagles, black crowned night herons, sand hill cranes, great blue herons, fox, coyote, deer, pheasant, hawks of various kinds, orioles, blue birds, scarlet tanagers, Jenny wrens, cedar wax wings, screech owls, great horned owls, grosbeaks, turkey, humming birds, downy woodpeckers, sap suckers, yellow bellied woodpeckers, frogs, toads, snakes bunnies, mink, voles and mice. Knowing they were all there made me feel less alone and for a moment I tapped their strength. If our farm could provide a living sanctuary for all of that wildlife, it most certainly could do the same for me. A surge of energy flowed through me and once again I grabbed ahold of life instead of death.

June 25, 2006
Staying on the plus side of life was a constant challenge. One day I was up and the next I was down. The next down came from three very important dot tattoos. While I lay on the radiation simulation bed, the radiation technician took a bottle of India ink in his left hand and squeezed the dropper to release one little drip onto my skin. He then, poked a needle into the middle of the drip providing a pathway for the ink to settle just under my skin. He wiped the excess ink away and then repeated the procedure two more times before helping me up. He explained that each spot was a permanent mark placed to guide the linear accelerator while it delivered high energy radiation to the tumor area

each day for 37 consecutive business days. It was unimaginable that I could muster the strength to trudge my way to those appointments day after day, but I did while embracing the help of the tiny voice of reason that popped up on my shoulder, pointing out that I had already gone through so much already. It only made sense to go all the way, otherwise the non-stop suffering would've been for naught. So on the morning of my first burn, I drove to the cancer center, walked through the glass doors and turned right at the front desk towards the radiation department instead of left to the chemo treatment area.

In the hall of the radiation wing, Nurse Ann was waiting to greet me with a cotton medical gown.

As she led me to the dressing room, she instructed, "Go ahead and put the gown on and wait here for me to come and get you. It shouldn't be long at all."

I did as I was told and sat alone in the long cotton gown patterned with flowers, closing my eyes to take in the silence. I was learning to love being alone and took advantage of the opportunity to visualize myself healthy and pray for strength. Barely breaking the silence, an older gentleman in a blue cotton medical gown falling to his knees slowly passed me on his way into the men's dressing room. We glanced at each other but didn't say word. There was no need.

Moments later, Nurse Ann arrived sweeping her right arm from the front of her body to the side and in a sing songy voice said, "All set for you, Kathy!"

I followed Ann into the cold and sterile radiation room. She dropped back behind me as I crossed the threshold, and when I turned to seek her direction, the thick metal door she stood beside took me completely by surprise. It was as thick as a concrete block and looked like the door of a bank vault without the locking mechanism. Ann swept her arm from front to back again encouraging me to move towards a cream-colored robot like machine where she asked me to disrobe and lay on the table. There were three technicians in all, and as I stared up at the ceiling, they each moved silently around me, performing their own choreographed tasks, tucking foam supports here and there under my body and placing a thin blanket over the parts of my body that would not be radiated.

When their movement stopped, I heard Ann through the speaker asking me to, "Breathe calmly. Stay as still as you can but go ahead and breathe normally."

The deep hum of the machine switched on, followed by the scuffling of technicians' feet bolting for the door and pulling it tight behind them. The hefty door was meant to contain any radiation overspray, and when it was sealed

133

shut, it seemed to suck the air out of the room all together. Although I couldn't see the door from my table, I knew I was alone amidst the imposing machines and spent a minute thinking about what it all meant. Without moving my head, I rolled my eyes to the right and then to the left, taking in my limited surroundings. The frigid, tiled room was lined by machines and cabinets filled with medical devices set next to foam pillows of different shapes and sizes, which were used to make patients like me more comfortable. I noted four empty spaces on the shelves where the pieces presently tucked around my body were stored. Looking for something positive to think about, I started with "It was nice that they thought about that," and ended with "but comfort while submitting to cancer killing doses of radiation is hard to find."

As the machine moved around me, I succumbed to the third stage of my recovery and tumbled into a peaceful nap, counting on meditation to carry me through. Having given up my regular practice in exchange for pity, I was surprised to find I could still conjure a meditative state that liberated me from the shackles of my physical limitations.

July 4, 2006
On the 4th of July, Ron packed our day full of hiking, swimming for the girls (wading for me) and dinner out with friends. Unfortunately, I lost my grip on peace and flipped.

"I can't do this! I'm exhausted! Why won't you just let me sleep?" I yelled at Ron.

"I'm sorry. I thought you'd want to get out of the house. I'm sorry. I won't schedule anything else. I was just trying to be helpful." Ron quietly replied.

He was right, of course. It was better for all of us to get out of the house, especially the girls. I just couldn't be normal because I didn't feel normal, and I was acutely aware that I wasn't normal and was in all ways slower. I couldn't find the words I wanted to say and had trouble following conversations because the constant chatter was too much for me to process. My feet shuffled instead of taking the long purposeful strides of my cancer free days. In the end, I agreed to go, trying to participate in the festivities but failing miserably.

"Please. Can we go home. I really can't do this. I need to go home," I pleaded with Ron before dinner.

His exasperated sigh ushered in pity as he responded, "Sure. You go to the car, and I'll collect the girls. I'll make a bonfire on the drumlin, and we can watch the fireworks from there."

The girls loved hilltop bonfires, so any disappointment they might've felt about not swimming any longer, shimmered off and morphed into expectant delight. On our way home, Ron purchased four plastic chairs at the hardware store on which he invited the girls to write their names with black Sharpie while he lit the fire. Since Hannah hadn't learned to write, EmmaGrace did the honors and instead of writing our real names, she wrote "Papa Bear," "Mama Bear," "Baby Hannah Bear" and "Goldilocks EmmaGrace Bear." While she finished her task, Hannah ran around each chair laughing and goading her big sister to hurry up so they could play. Throughout the remainder of the evening, they picked prairie flowers, chased each other, stood on a stump and sang at the top of their lungs, howled for the coyotes, and then collapsed into their new chairs next to the blazing fire. A few clouds passed through the dusk sprinkling us with a light rain, which revealed a very bright rainbow still visible in the darkening sky. EmmaGrace ran off to find the pot of gold she was so certain was there, and I took its vibrancy as a sign that everything would be all right.

The lightening bugs emerged like stars amidst the prairie grasses swishing in the light evening breeze. Noticing my closed eyes and bobbing head, the girls urged me to stay awake for the fireworks. From our vantage point, we could see 15 different displays within a 180-degree view. There was no traffic to battle, no crowds to work around and an unending supply of s'mores. It was the perfect way to celebrate Independence Day. I searched for some sort of symbolism or larger meaning for myself and settled in on my own corny phrasing that it was "Independence From Cancer Day." I constantly looked for meaning in everything back then, which I blamed on the culture of cancer counselling. Sometimes, an event was just an event and nothing more.

July 9, 2006
As the days marched on, it became almost impossible for me to do anything other than go to my radiation treatments and take care of the girls in the afternoon. I thought radiation would be easier but it wasn't. With little time to regroup and gain strength after chemo and surgery, it became just another sledgehammer beating me down. I was beyond exhausted, which left me defenseless against the nausea, headaches and pain of burning skin.

My mom visited as much as possible, and her arrival at the house heralded the brief departure of cancer's oppressive cloud, making way for effortless play and laughter for my girls. For me, it meant the pressure to entertain two wonderfully energetic girls was off my shoulders for the day. EmmaGrace and Hannah were always elated when my mom appeared. She was loads of fun and full of non-judgmental love. When they were annoyingly wild, she just laughed much like her mother had done with me when I was their age. Normally, I would hug her and thank her before disappearing into my room for a nap. When I reappeared in the mix, my mom would drive us to the top of the hill to take in the stunning array of colors blooming across the prairie. The landscape was beautiful with the orange of butterfly weed vivid against the back drop of pink coneflowers and purple prairie clover perfectly accented by the yellow cup plants towering over the white balls of the rattlesnake master. I would move into the dense prairie and stand amongst its dazzling colors, soaking in its fresh fragrant air while the girls ran through the fields picking bouquets.

Later that day, we all drove to my radiation appointment. It wasn't something my mom did with any regularity, and I couldn't have known how grateful I would be to have her there that particular day because after my radiation treatment, Dr. Arnold led me to his office and reported exactly what I didn't want to hear. He believed I would require more treatments than what he had originally planned. I collapsed. My armpit was raw, bloody and painful. I had to hold my right arm slightly off to the side in an effort to reduce the painful friction, which only served to create more problems in my shoulder joint and neck. I was in a constant battle of weighing which pain was worse and choosing the lesser of two evils.

"You see what's happening to my skin. How can I possibly take anymore?" I asked sincerely, wanting an answer, but he gave me no reply.

After my appointment, my mom drove the girls and I to the local bookstore, attempting to switch my frame of focus. Both girls loved books and our little Books & Company was strategically placed next to the coffee shop. My mom directed me to the comfy chairs in the children's section and got each of us a cup of coffee next door. Then, she plunked herself down into the chair next to mine. I sipped in the soothing warmth of some sort of blend while the girls picked book after book off the shelves, holding them up for me to see.

"Look at this one!" EmmaGrace whisper shouted.

"I like this one!" Hannah said following her big sister's lead.

All I had to do was smile.

My mom took over all responses with, "Ooooo, that looks like a good one. I really like the title!"

After almost a full hour, the girls came to me with their arms full of books, asking if I would buy them all. I laughed and held up two fingers. As they dropped to the floor to evaluate their choices, I glanced at my mom who was smiling lovingly at me. I knew how special I was to her, but I wondered if she knew just how special she was to me. I smiled back and told her I loved her.

July 15, 2006
My dad came out to the house to have lunch with the girls and me. He struggled with wanting to do something more not realizing his visits were enough. He brought flowers for me and books for the girls.

"I wish I had cancer so I could get flowers," EmmaGrace said with a huge grin.

I looked at my dad and swallowed hard. Neither one of us knew what to say to that. I hugged him and told him he was the best dad ever. He cared so deeply and was never afraid to express his love. He enjoyed each and every one of us without condition. My dad always found something to appreciate in most people, but his love of and patience with kids was something I had seen in few men. I remembered one particular day when I was a kid and my Grandpa was over helping my dad build a screened-in porch with me and my siblings hanging all over him and getting in the way.

"How can you take this?" my Grandpa asked my Dad.

"I love them. I'd rather have them happy and wanting to be with me than moody and distant," he responded as if his answer should've been obvious.

It was as if he was actually asking my Grandpa, "why wouldn't you?"

July 17, 2006
Hilltop fires had become the activity of choice for my little family. As Ron drove us up, I prayed that a noise proof shell would magically appear around my chair, leaving me to watch the action in my own peaceful little bubble. As I got out of the truck, the girls surrounded me elated to let loose without the constraints of indoor play. Recognizing my frightened expression, Ron yelled with an attack dog type of growl that made me cringe. They quickly quieted down and moved their play away for me, giving me a chance to get to my chair. As soon as I sat, they were right back, singing, dancing and falling into me with hugs and kisses, forcing me to deflect their outpouring of affection away from my charred torso. The coyotes in the den behind our hill joined in, and their howls made everyone laugh but me.

"I have to go to bed now. I love you guys," I said with feigned enthusiasm and stumbled my way back down the hill to our house with the mournful sounds of the coyotes following me the entire way.

I normally loved to hear them sing, but on that night, I fell into the front door and cried out loud, "How could being loved hurt so much? When would it all end? I can't even be around my family anymore!"

July 18, 2006
I welcomed what I hoped would be a good day at the cancer clinic, and it was. The radiation oncologist had decided I didn't need additional treatments. It was surreal. The plan never seemed to work in my favor. I was at the point where nothing the cancer center gave me to relieve the pain worked, and I couldn't comprehend how I could possibly endure any more. Once again, Suzannah came to my rescue, procuring a prescription for silver sulfadiazine, an antibiotic paste with lidocaine developed for burn victims and used widely at Memorial Sloan-Kettering. I slathered the white paste all over my burned skin and used a thick bandage of cooling gel to keep it from rubbing off on my clothes. The pain faded to a dull vibration, which was just enough of a reprieve to restore my faith that there would come a day when I would suffer no longer.

July 20, 2006
Hannah and I dropped EmmaGrace at Brownie camp, then ran some errands. I explained to her that we were buying things to get ready for our vacation. Apparently, we hadn't described our previous trip to Colorado as a vacation, so she had no idea what the word meant. I had a moment of panic wondering what else I had neglected to teach her. I held up my left hand to show her the shape of Wisconsin and pointed to my thumb, describing it as Door County, a favored destination for many. Then I used my index finger to motion a dot in the air above my thumb.

"That's where we're going. Washington Island," I told her. "So, today we're buying some odds and ends that we might not be able to get there."

Hannah didn't respond or ask any more questions until we were home and I was unbuckling her car seat.

She gave me a confused look and asked, "Were we on vacation?"

"No, Honey. We were ORGANIZING for vacation." I said kissing her forehead but wanting to squeeze her tighter than I ever had before.

I giggled out loud and was promptly punished by a nauseating, stabbing pain. It reflected the constant emotional conflict I confronted nearly every day. I left the bags behind for Ron to unload, put Hannah down for a nap and went to my room to free my bloody skin. The radiation burn covered an area under my right arm, across the right side of my chest and onto the inside of my left breast. As I

138

took a deep breath in, the inevitable surge of dread erupted, prickling my skin from the inside out. Taking the left hand corner of the bandage, I held it firmly, lifting carefully so it wouldn't drop back down, then gently pulled it up and off to my right side before tossing it in the garbage. I sat slumped on my bed, waiting for the return of my bravery and then slathered the silver sulfadiazine over every bit of red area on my blistering and bleeding chest. The pain was excruciating, growing worse with every treatment, and attempting to avert my attention from my own agony, I pictured the myriad burn victims suffering far worse than I. Crying for them or maybe for myself, I dropped into bed and slept the rest of the afternoon.

My last day of radiation was July 28, 2006. It was a Thursday and by the weekend my chest was a mess. The third-degree burns were streaming red, yellow and clear fluids constantly throughout the day and night. When I tried to apply the burn cream, it just slipped around unable to take hold. When I pleaded with my doctors to do something about it, they were even surprised by the degree of charring on my body. No one knew how to help me and by the following Monday, I was lost in anguish.

My skin was gone. The radiation had burned it off, leaving me to writhe in bed, drowning in high doses of morphine, which failed to do anything more than take the edge off. Finding no relief in bed and with clothing completely out of the question, I draped myself in a lightweight cotton sheet and paced. Just like food in a microwave, I felt myself roasting moment by moment from the inside out. The doctors erred on the side of increasing my morphine dose, which didn't touch the actual pain but left me distressingly disoriented. In my silence, a little voice encouraged me to choose pain over confusion, and without questioning that notion, I tossed the drugs into the garbage before the next one was due. In that exact second, somewhere deep inside my soul, the imperative to hug my girls took hold with absolute urgency. I secured the sheet and scuffled quickly down the stairs once again certain that death was on my heels. I had to tell them how much I loved them before the reaper overtook my ravaged body. They were playing with tinker toys and I asked EmmaGrace for a kiss, which she was glad to give. Then, I did the same with Hannah who studied me in dismay.

She scolded, "Mommy, you put on too much lotion."

I called Suzannah and begged her to rescue me, which she did of course. She created a new routine for me using Ultram ER and 600 mg of Ibuprofen taken orally throughout the day. Then, I applied silver sulfadiazine, covered it with Vigilon and wrapped the whole area in Kerlex. At night, I used Lansinoh, softening the paste as it warmed between my fingers. It was summer and the temperature outside was approaching 100 degrees each and every day. I was forced to stay indoors with the air conditioning set to 60 degrees, pacing like a caged lion with a railroad spike thrust into my collarbone and chest. It was excruciating.

Ron and I decided to accept offers from our mothers to take the girls over the following week. I thanked God for them daily. Each day the radiation continued its work, burning new areas adjacent to the target zone, but Suzannah's program did seem to help, if only by providing me some sort of rhythm.

August 1, 2006
Although I still wasn't healed, the pain was finally tolerable and I looked forward to our Island escape. While Ron packed the car, I carefully wrapped up my chest and put on an oversized shirt before making my way to the car to sit delicately in the front seat. I reached for the seat belt, realizing I couldn't put it across my chest and settled in to resting my elbow on the door while holding the belt just off my body. Determined to stay positive, I opened my air conditioning vent to full blast and perched on the seat braced for the five-hour drive. When we arrived at the tip of Door County in a tiny village called Gilles Rock, we turned right towards Northport, which had nothing more than an abandoned restaurant and a dock. We drove across the dock and onto the Washington Island Ferry where we parked. The girls jumped out of the car and climbed the stairs up to the open-air deck. I wanted to join them, but as soon as they opened the car doors, a stifling heat was ushered in. I turned the car back on and blasted the air conditioning once again, expecting to feel sad but actually found myself smiling. I felt happy, genuinely happy, and caught just a glimpse of what life was like before I was labeled a cancer patient. It was enough to dim the pain for a little while and give me hope that the end of my misery was near.

Within the hour, we were off the ferry and in our home away from home. One of my friends had given us the keys to her island get away filled with all the amenities except one. Of all the things her cabin could've been missing, the worst for me was an air conditioner. I panicked, fruitlessly searching the walls for a dial.

"Ron! I can't find any way to turn the air conditioning on. Why can't I find the dial?!" I called.

In a flash, Ron investigated around the outside of the house before reporting back that there indeed was no air conditioner. I stood in disbelief while he scurried past me, opening all of the windows and turning on a fan for me to sit in front of. It was enough.

The next day, we hung out at the most popular beach on the island - School House Beach. It wasn't a typical sandy beach. It was filled with smooth white limestone rocks unique to the bay. Unfortunately the day was simply too hot for me, so I sat in the air conditioned car

while Ron and the girls played in the water. Instead of grumbling, I used my time to reconnect with my meditation practice and visualization skills, imagining my chest healed and the cancer gone. I did that multiple times a day, and noticed that as the week went on a little bit of new skin inched its way over the open wound. Was it coincidence? At first, the growth was imperceptible, but as the end of the week approached, it was clear that new skin was indeed growing and had completely closed the wound. I was able to wear normal clothes and stood in the lake while the girls splashed around me. Each passing day brought less and less pain, allowing me to drop the pain medication all together, which proved to be a big mistake. I had become physically addicted. Mentally, I didn't want to take it anymore, but my body craved it. I anxiously paced the cabin, finding sleep elusive. Ron called Suzannah who confirmed that I was absolutely in withdrawal and would need to go back on to phase off properly. She described a new schedule for me and it wasn't long before I had control of my body once again.

August 13, 2006
With the burns almost completely healed, fatigue took center stage. By mid-morning, it felt like an imaginary gauze sheet was thrown over my head. My brain function grew fuzzy and before too long, the gauze transformed into a heavy, dark, velvet drape, collapsing on me as I fell into the nearest couch. I couldn't fight it. My fractured ribs made it painful to breathe and pain shot from the mediport scar up along the left side of my neck to the back of my ear. On top of it all, I contracted a bladder infection and called Mary immediately. She sent a prescription for antibiotics to the drug store and Ron picked them up on his way home. I was always deeply appreciative of how my cancer center made life as easy as possible for me, especially Mary.

I was sitting on a kitchen chair when Hannah appeared by my side to say, "You're my Mommy. I love you!" then dropped down for a very long hug, demanding me to stay strong.

Later that week, I decided to step on the scale in my quest for some positive news. To my utter shock, the weight loss I was aiming for suddenly flipped and I had gained 10 pounds in the blink of an eye.

Devastated, I called Dr. Tousignant who said with heartfelt compassion, "It's most likely because of the Zoloft, but you need to stay on it for one year.

141

Then, you should be out of the woods with the side effects of menopause."

I found no real comfort in her words because gaining 10 pounds was entirely counter to my health goals. From the perspective of my doctors it wasn't anything to worry about, but fat cells produced hormones which the cancer loved to grab hold of, and I couldn't afford to give it any help. Aromasin or not the fat had to go. During an appointment with Dr. Sanders to discuss the final phase of my breast reconstruction, I asked him to liposuction my fat away. It was something I never would've considered while I was healthy, but after everything I had been through, it only seemed fair that I should get a little help in that department. He agreed, but in a scolding voice told me it wasn't a license to gain more weight, as if I had any control over my body at all.

"Keep your weight down. I can only safely take so much out at one time," he cautioned. "You also need to understand that taking the fat cells out of one area of your body means you can gain fat somewhere else."

Admittedly, I didn't understand what that meant until several years later when I realized my upper arms were bigger and I had developed fat on my back. I couldn't say the trade-off was worth it, but then again, hind sight was always 20/20.

August 20, 2006
Once I was healed enough to give hugs, the girls gave them all the time with EmmaGrace becoming an enthusiastic hugger once again.

One night, she ran to me and said, "I just want to kiss you every time I see you, Mommy!"

Hannah snuggled in bed with me and said, "Your owie is gone. You're better, MaMa!"

Then Hannah got a sad face looking around the room for the flowers.

"They're all gone," I told her. "They gave me all their energy, so I could get better."

Hannah squeezed me hard, and I could feel her smile against my skin. I took that loving period in time to write them a note, which I tucked away in my journal for when they were older.

> *"Hi, Girls!*
> *If you're reading this, please know how much I love you both*

for who you are. I couldn't have made it through these last 10 months without your laughter and love. It was for the two of you that I fought so hard, piling on the assault to my cancer. The doctors couldn't believe that I never took a break from my treatment and my response is always the same, 'How could I? I have babies.' I've always known I gather strength in the face of a crisis, but now I can say it unequivocally, I am strong because of you two.

If this cancer ends up taking me, just know that I left no stone unturned. I fought with the help of my doctors, Aunt Suzannah and all our family. There were lots of people praying for me and I prayed all throughout the day. Don't ever abandon your faith. It will sustain you in times of need, bring a smile to your face in times of joy and comfort you in times of confusion.

EmmaGrace and Hannah, stay strong, tough and brave. Love yourselves and each other. Love yourselves and your families enough to face any challenge life throws your way, and recognize it as an opportunity to grow. Sometimes the spoils aren't clear, but good comes out of every difficultly we face whether we win or lose. I love you both in a way words can never convey."

August 28, 2006

Time was ticking by. I still spent a lot of time lying down on the couch with Hannah by my side. She hugged me often, sang to me and twirled around sometimes grabbing my hand to dance with her. Her healing presence astounded me. From the couch, I enjoyed the entertainment Hannah provided, and soaked up the warmth I felt when she squeezed me tightly, pressing her cheek against mine. One day, she twirled over to me and placed her hand on my arm. I felt a jolt or spark of energy transfer from her to me. It was a warm and comforting sensation travelling up my arm and through my body and felt absolutely surreal and real at the same time.

Hannah bounced off me and went back to twirling while she sang, "I just healed you, Mommy!"

And it truly felt like she had.

Unfortunately, one of the things Hannah hadn't healed was my memory. Another side effect of the prescription drug cocktail not listed anywhere on their fact sheets was memory loss. There was so much I didn't remember and so much I remembered incorrectly when relying solely on my memory bank.

Luckily, my cancer counselors at Stillwaters encouraged me to keep a journal. Making regular entries throughout my experience had allowed me to hold details more accurately than my memory ever could have. While the physical side-effects were the focus of the medical community, I was struggling intellectually as well. Conversations were more difficult and my cognitive challenges became almost crippling. On occasion when I'd try to join a conversation with other parents at school, I'd notice their annoyance. It seemed that what my brain wanted to say was not what my tongue released from my lips. Too often my conversations were scattered with irrelevant statements, leaving me feeling embarrassed and pathetic. At our small private school, EmmaGrace and I were being pushed aside. A cancer diagnosis is a call to action for most, but sustaining that support reaches a limit. The parents at our school seemed to tire of the whole affair. The dinners from the early months were less frequent and I felt like my cancer battle had become "so yesterday."

September 14, 2006
The television offered comfort on some days and distress on others. One day, I plopped myself down in front of the television to watch the news, and the story being reported threw me for a complete loop. The reporter was interviewing a mother who had lost her daughter to inflammatory breast cancer. The daughter was quite a bit younger than I was, and when the first signs of the disease appeared on her breast, her doctor misdiagnosed the red spot as a spider bite. By the time he got her diagnosis right, the aggressive cancer had spread. That poor woman fought for two years before succumbing, and I couldn't help but note that I was just about to hit the one year mark. Oddly enough, I believed with my entire being that I would live and yet, found myself questioning that belief because it wasn't true for others.

I switched my focus from the negative to the positive and decided to take EmmaGrace for a walk in the woods. She was so curious about everything, searching the leaf litter for something interesting to examine. Almost immediately she found yellowish green fungi the size of volleyballs clinging to the forest floor. She wondered with amazement at them while I reminded her that they were called giant puffballs just like the ones we found in our front yard the previous year.

"These are older versions of the ones we found. Remember? They were white and I cut them up and fried them in the skillet?" I asked questioning her long-term memory.

"I think so," she said unsure if she remembered eating something so gross.

"These are a different color because they are almost spent. If we stomp on them, a puff of yellow dust will come out. Those are the spores, something like seeds, that they send out to make new puffballs next year," I explained.

"Can I step on one?" she asked.

"Yeah! Let's do it!" I exclaimed.

For the next 45 minutes, we jumped, stomped and squished puffballs all through the forest floor, making our final act to leave our footprint on the biggest ones we could find. As we admired the impressions, EmmaGrace took my hand, causing my heart to burst with joy. She held on the whole way home and we ended our little adventure, snuggled on the couch like we used to do.

Sweet moments like those usually didn't last long because they always seemed to give way to some new problem. Next up were debilitating headaches accompanied by severe abdominal pain. I unsuccessfully tried to find relief in meditation before calling Suzannah who instructed me to take ibuprofen or acetaminophen.

"If the pain goes away, then it's not likely to be from cancer. A cancer headache is typically present at all times of the day. If it goes away, it's probably from anxiety," she explained sounding confident.

I took some ibuprofen and the pain subsided.

September 29, 2006
Ron flew to Montana for work, leaving me both nervous and empowered at the prospect of taking care of the girls by myself. I hadn't done that in almost an entire year and it felt exhilarating. Unfortunately, I woke up that first morning dizzy and unable to keep my balance. I immediately called Dr. Harper who ordered me into the hospital for an MRI. The girls were just waking up and I needed to get them to school first, so I slid down the hall bracing myself against the wall as I made my way to EmmaGrace's room.

"I need your help, Honey. I need you to get Hannah up and get both

of you ready for school. I'll be in the kitchen trying to get your breakfast ready," I said as calmly as I could.

Beyond that, I don't remember a thing except intense pain in my ear and pressure in my head. Through divine intervention, I got them to school and me to the hospital, although I have no memory of how. I remembered waking EmmaGrace up and then nothing until I was in the mobile MRI unit behind the hospital. The rest is unrecoverable. Clearly, my guardian angel took over because there is no other plausible explanation. The results of the MRI came back immediately, revealing that I had another tumor in my head and neck

145

primarily in the parotid gland, a major salivary gland next to my left ear. The mass was putting pressure on my eustachian tube, which was the source of my pain and loss of balance. The Ear Nose and Throat (ENT) doctor on duty recommended immediate surgery. His name was Dr. Petri, and he explained that the surgery was tantamount to a partial face-lift. He went on to explain the gruesome details of peeling back part of my face to remove the lump. He gave me Sudafed to relieve the pressure in my ear, and when I recovered my balance, I abruptly took my leave and made a bee line for Dr. Harper's office. While he appeared calm, it was hard to miss his irritation with Dr. Petri. After a quick exam, he sent me to another ENT Dr. Fredrick who recommended a biopsy to assess what they were dealing with. Ron cut his meetings short and flew home the next day, trying to comfort me the only way he knew how.

"It's going to be fine," he said.

I exploded, "It's not fine! None of this is fine! I can't take anymore, and if you tell me I'm going to be fine one more time, I don't know what I'll do! I AM CLEARLY NOT FINE!"

"I'm sorry. I just don't know what to say. I'm so sad for you. It's terrible you have to go through so much and it doesn't seem to ever end."

I was grateful for his honesty and capitalized on the moment, "Would you please go and talk to a cancer counselor?"

He agreed.

I breathed.

October 12, 2006
Janet drove me to the Waukesha Memorial Hospital and walked me to the outpatient department. I was there to have a biopsy of the tumor behind my ear and was terrified. After I checked in, Janet hugged me before they split us up, sending her to the waiting room and me to yet another procedure room. I don't remember the doctor's name, having forgotten to write it in my notebook. I supposed I was trying to distance myself from what was about to happen.

Once I was on the table the nurse asked, "Would you mind if we lighten the mood."

I immediately felt the call to action and flipped my attitude, "Be my guest! I've made it through inflammatory breast cancer treatment. I can handle this too, so

146

bring it on!"

We all laughed and then the procedure began. While I couldn't see what the doctor was doing, it felt like he was chiseling away at my bone. The sound was gritty, like a shovel jabbing into very tightly packed sand or a bed of tiny pebbles. Thanks to the Lidocaine shot I only felt pressure until the biopsy needle hit my ear canal. I jumped and the doctor immediately pulled it out, asking if I was all right. Not waiting for an answer, he smiled and left the room to have the pathologist look at the sample.

When he returned, he said, "We have good news. The cells look very different from the breast cancer cells, so it's not metastasized breast cancer, but it is cancer. We'll get the pathology results back in two days, so for now you're free to go and run out the door as fast as you want. I won't take it personally."

October 14, 2006

I was resting on the couch when Dr. Fredrick called with the results of my biopsy. My chest felt tight and sharp pains materialized in my gut. Whether I wanted to believe it or not, I had another cancer diagnosis.

"It is a tumor and it needs to come out," Dr. Fredrick reported to me.

"What is it?" I asked expecting her to say it was in fact metastasized breast cancer.

"It's a mucoepidermoid carcinoma. With this type of cancer, we need to know the grade to decide what kind of treatment to give you. We can more reliably do that after we've taken it out. I'll need you to talk with my assistant to get your appointments organized. Don't worry. It's not a bad cancer. We'll take care of it," she said with the utmost confidence.

Later that same day, Milwaukee Fox 6 News interviewed Suzannah and me. The reporter Julie was doing a story on inflammatory breast cancer. There weren't a lot of patients with that particular cancer, and I had agreed to talk with her when I thought my battle was over. With the new diagnosis, I almost cancelled, but Suzannah encouraged me to go ahead with it. We met Julie at Suzannah's house and she immediately commented about how I "was so matter of fact" with all of my answers. I wasn't sure what she meant by that, wondering if she wanted me to break down and cry on camera. I wanted to unleash the anger and frustration I was carrying at that moment but didn't and settled on just being rude.

"Why are you surprised and impressed by my control? It's a weird thing to say to someone like me," I asked unapologetically.

Her eyes were soft and her voice dropped to almost a whisper, "my husband's first wife died of breast cancer and now I'm raising her 13-year-old daughter. I just think it must be impossible for you to manage everything with two small girls."

I was humbled.

October 20, 2006

I gained weight no matter what I did and was embarrassed that my previously athletic body was more like the Pillsbury Dough Boy. With my recovery plan stalled and displaced by removing a new tumor, I went to Kohl's Department Store and bought a pair of pants the next size up, then finished my day giving more blood for pre-surgical screening. With every surgery, my blood seemed to be tested in different ways, and for the parotidectomy, they wanted to know where my thyroid was at. There was no explanation why they were testing it, but I was so glad they had. My TSH was 85, an incredibly high number, signifying permanent damage to my thyroid as a result of the aggressive radiation I had undergone. I was diagnosed with "hypothyroidism" and was thrilled to finally have a partial answer for my growing waist. The high TSH number meant that my thyroid wasn't producing enough hormone to effectively run my metabolism, but with one small oval shaped pill called Levothyroxine that was easily corrected. So, Levothyroxine was assigned the task of getting my metabolism back on track and hopefully helping me shed some weight.

I recalled my sister-in-law Jo labeling her own hypothyroidism and calling it out like a cheer, "Hypo=Hippo!"

The newly discovered tumor was scheduled to be resected on October 26, 2006, one day shy of the one year anniversary of my original diagnosis. Clearly, there would be no celebrating as I welcomed the wagons circling around me once again. There were slight differences in who drove them, however, with my friend Lisa taking the reins on one of them. She called to tell me she had spoken to her brother, an ENT in Colorado, who urged me to have my surgery done by Dr. Harrison at the University of Wisconsin-Madison Carbone Cancer Center. Lisa's brother believed he was the best otolaryngologist in the country and since he was less than an hour from my house, it didn't make any sense to go to someone else. The bonus with Dr. Harrison was that he was also a plastic surgeon, which meant scarring would

be negligible. Lisa's brother offered to get me an appointment right away and I graciously agreed, embracing the new team taking over my care if only for a little while.

Suzannah was my companion and personal advocate at that first appointment in Madison, helping me translate Dr. Harrison's analysis of my situation. He explained that the intricacies of my tumor were more complicated than I had been led to believe. He laid out the pros and cons of him doing my surgery, with the only con being that his hospital was an hour from my family. Since that really wasn't an issue for us, he said a cordial good bye and let his team take over scheduling my surgery. After I signed the requisite papers, Suzannah led me through the waiting room and across the all to the breast center for our previously agreed to appointment with Dr. Stevenson who was reviewing my case to recommend follow-up care.

Dr. Stevenson was a quick study. His demeanor was kind and respectful as he expressed sadness at all that I had been through before shifting to an optimistic outlook for my prognosis.

"I think it's a good idea for you to stay on Aromasin. If the cancer comes back, we'll have new chemotherapies to try. Treatments are just improving all the time, and I was pleased to read that you added Avastin in the mix. It's looking like an excellent option for my patients." Dr. Stevenson said. "I really think you're prognosis looks good, but I would not like to see you do too much more by way of post screening. I recommend a physical exam every two to three months and a mammogram every other year. I'm just afraid if we keep scanning you, we're going to give you more cancer."

"What about my parotid surgery? Could my doctor at home do it or is Dr. Harrison better?" I asked.

Dr. Stevenson chose his words carefully as he got up from his chair to end our appointment, "Why don't I call Dr. Harper and discuss it with him. I whole-heartedly agree with your friend's brother that Dr. Harrison is the best."

I marveled at his efficiency in thoroughly answering every one of our question while still expressing compassion for my situation. I packed up my file as he waited at the door to lead us out, and Suzannah took advantage of the opportunity to point out the need for patient advocates, which was not a thing in Wisconsin when I was diagnosed.

Suzannah commented, "Having cancer really requires a full-time secretary for each patient. There is so much involved, and it's difficult to keep it all straight, if you don't know what you're doing."

149

"That's for sure," Dr. Stevenson agreed.

October 22, 2006
The daily pain in my ear expanded wrapping itself around my head and becoming more intense with every passing day. My neck muscles ached and my ears rang off the hook.

I called Dr. Harrison and pleaded for answers, "What's going on? Why does it hurt so much more than it did last week?"

"It probably means the tumor is changing," he said more calmly than I thought he should have sounded.

Waves of terror swept over me as I imagined where the tumor might be moving to.

"Could it be going into my brain," I asked with fearful urgency.

"I highly doubt it," Dr. Harrison coolly responded. "It's more likely that the tumor is wrapping itself more tightly around a nerve. If it's around the wrong nerve, you could suffer long-term damage to your face, but that hasn't happened to any of my patients yet."

When I hung up the phone, I prayed with renewed intensity that the surgery to peel back my ear and scalp would be simple, and I would recover without complication. I was ready to be normal again and didn't know how much more I could take. I drew from Dr. Harrison's composed demeanor and tried to relax into the next step along my path. Unfortunately as is often the case with research hospitals, my surgery was postponed for more than two weeks. Managing the pain was harder every day and I almost couldn't remember what it was like to live pain free. I knew I couldn't afford self-defeating thoughts, so I was left with no choice but to build a wall around my negativity and stay focused on my clearly defined job to fight cancer. I shifted my word choices to weaken its hold on me, referring to the new tumor as more of an annoyance. The more I said it out loud, the more I believed it and the better I felt. However once night fell and I lay in bed, the façade faded away and my mind focused mercilessly on the potential surgical damage to my facial nerve. If Dr. Harrison couldn't work around it, one side of my face would become paralyzed.

October 29, 2006
It was Halloween again and my energy was too low for trick-or-treating, but there was no way the girls were going to miss out. So Ron and I devised a plan for them to trick-or-treat at our house. I got the girls dressed in their costumes,

handed them each a pumpkin shaped bucket and instructed them to run from door to door being careful not to miss one. They wasted no time and ran enthusiastically around the house while I tried to keep up, moving from door to door with candy tray in hand, feigning surprise with each knock. Laughter truly was the best medicine that night, relegating that mass growing in my head to not even an after-thought. When I ran out of candy, the girls busted through the back door, running to the family room where they dumped their orange, plastic Jack-O-Lantern out to admire the sugar load before them. I watched with happy memories of doing the same with my own siblings as we traded up for our favorite candy. My parents watched us just as I was watching my girls learn a little something about the negotiation process while I learned a little more about what was most valuable in their haul. For example, EmmaGrace traded two Skittle bags for one Air Head.

October 31, 2006
The new thyroid meds seemed to be working. In 10 days, four pounds had dropped from my weakening frame and I had a little more energy to work with. Unfortunately, the usual scenario of pleasant progress being over shadowed by negative news predictably played out once again. A simple yawn signaled a disturbing development. When I yawned, my eyebrow twitched uncomfortably. The muscle seemed to stick and then go flat, clearly demonstrating that the nerve was indeed involved. I grabbed a deep breath, looked up to the heavens and instead of calling Dr. Harrison in a panic, I meditated.

After 20 mins or so, I decreed, "What will be will be."

November 11, 2006
The headache Suzannah had described previously had arrived. It was there every day all day and was difficult to ignore. I spent my time moving around the house doing laundry, cleaning, organizing and yelling at the kids. The medication brought anger even I was afraid of. If the tumor wasn't altering my brain function, the medication surely was. It was impossible to stop myself as the horrifying words came spewing out followed by an almost instant apology to the girls.

"Oh my gosh! I'm so sorry. That was completely out of line," I said expressing deep regret.

"It's OK, Mama. I know you don't mean it," EmmaGrace answered with gracious forgiveness.

"No. It's not OK. It's never OK for someone to talk to you like that. I have no idea what's happening to me with these medications," I asserted, fearing that

151

she would grow up thinking it was normal for people to yell at each other.

November 12, 2006
With surgery only one day away, I let the answering machine catch the stream of calls offering support and opted to express my appreciation via email. While I initially welcomed the wagons, I felt like I needed to say, "There's nothing to see here, Folks. You can all go home." My thoughts were pulled to the potential results of a paralyzed face, and meditation seemed like the only way to push those fears aside. In an attempt to help me out, Ron brought home "Click," an Adam Sandler movie. His movies were often silly and Ron hoped it would lighten the mood in our house, but "Click" wasn't like the other Sandler movies. It carried a strong message about setting priorities.

When it concluded, Ron took my hand and said, "Let's move from here and find another house that needs work."

My response surprised even me.

I said in a relatively deadpan tone, "It's quite likely that I'll be dead in a couple years, and I don't want that time to be spent fixing up another house."

His response was equally as surprising, "Yeah, I know."

My attention turned to a scenario worse than death, and a new priority emerged. If I was to become incapacitated and unable to function on my own, I wanted to die. I didn't like the idea of machines keeping me alive with my family hanging around a hospice room waiting for the inevitable. My determination to be strong and vibrant created an overwhelming feeling deep in my soul. I felt myself revving up for some inevitable event, but each time I was about to "know" what it was, it slipped from my mind's eye view. It was impossible for me to know if it was death or some other task God had in store for me, but what I did know was both options brought me peace.

I fell asleep that night with this prayer, "Please let this be the end of cancer battles for me. I think I've proven myself to be brave, formidable, determined and strong. I will be victorious. I promise. So, can I be done now?"

November 13, 2006
My mom and dad drove to the hospital with us, and after I checked in at the University of Wisconsin – Madison Hospital and Clinics, my entourage escorted me to the pre-op area for surgical preparations. I tried to keep the mood light, but it wasn't easy in that solemn environment.

The pre-op nurse Laura ran through her standard questions. "When did you last eat? When did you last drink? What was it? What is your pain level on a scale from 0-10?"

Then, she left the curtained off space where I was lying on a gurney to tell Dr. Harrison I was ready. Moments later, Laura returned with the bad news that he had an emergency surgery, so mine would be delayed by more than two hours. We all gasped followed by her trying to recover the moment.

"Did you say you had a bad headache?" she asked.

"Yes. I didn't have any coffee this morning." I answered.

"How many cups do you drink each morning?" Laura asked.

"One or two," I answered.

"I'll be right back," she said turning away with a grin.

Moments later, she was back at my bedside wearing a huge smile and carrying a syringe filled with a clear liquid.

"What is that?" I asked.

"It's my secret weapon. It's caffeine. I'm going to give it to you through your IV and you're going to feel like a million bucks!" She said with such enthusiasm I had to believe her.

The plunger forced the caffeine into my IV tube and within seconds a cool wave moved across the front of my brain erasing the pain and bringing instant relief. Maybe I didn't feel like a million bucks, but I felt good enough to reach out and give my nurse a hug.

November 14, 2006
I made it through the surgery with my face intact, but my ear and jaw felt like a medieval ramming log had been repeatedly thrust into them. I was released the day after surgery, but I couldn't talk, chew or even swallow without intense pain. Even so, I didn't care. Dr. Harrison believed he had gotten all the cancer and was "almost" positive it wasn't a high-grade tumor, but we'd wait for the pathology report to confirm his impressions by the end of the week. At home Ron tucked me away in my bedroom where I could comfortably visit with my parents. They were noticeably relieved when they walked through the door, but I was surprised to see my dad, who under normal conditions would never show

153

up in my bedroom. He leaned in close to me and said he needed to give me a hug. I squeezed him as tightly as I could and Ron brought a chair in for my mom to sit next to my bed, holding my hand for quite some time and showering me in the electricity of her limitless love. There had never been a time when she was not available to me because she was always willing to give up anything for her kids. I never questioned where her priorities were. There I was at 42 still needing my mom, and there she was at 69 still holding my hand.

After my parents left and just before the kids went to bed, EmmaGrace came to my side and scolded me, "I am so mad at you, Mama. Why can't you be like the other moms? I had another dream last night that I was stabbing you."

In my mind, I ran through the things I wanted to say in response for example, "Look I am here. I am fighting as hard as I can to stay with you. Why can't you just love me? Why can't everyone just surround me with happy. I am suffering far more than any of you realize. I try not to show it because it will make you all uncomfortable, but I will get better. I promise."

Instead I said, "I'm mad too. I love you and know how hard this is for you. It will get better. I will get better because I am strong just like you."

November 16, 2006
I turned my prayers again to the scientists that worked so hard to find ways to make us better.

"God, please help the scientists stay on the side of doing what is right for humanity, not what will make big pharma the most money."

Dr. Harrison called with my results. He was wrong. The tumor was high-grade. The bad news was that I would be driving to Madison every day for some yet to be determined period of time to receive radiation therapy, but the good news was that I wouldn't have to have chemotherapy, and that was a silver lining worth noting. When I hung up, I couldn't stop the flood of tears and emotions swirling throughout my body and ejected them onto Ron like a bomb. My feelings had absolutely nothing to do with him, but I made them all about him.

"You're 'doing' everything that needs to be done, but you're not supporting me emotionally. All you're doing is pushing me further into loneliness and depression. Is that OK with you?" I blubbered noticing the intense pain building in my jaw.

Ron took a minute of silence and let loose, "You don't realize how hard it is for me. I'm dad, mom, breadwinner and caretaker. What else do you want me to do? I'm sad for you, but what else can I do? I'm exhausted!"

He was right. He had juggled so much to keep our lives moving along. He was more than a rock to our family, he was the whole planet. I don't know how he kept it all together. If I died, it would all be over for me, but he would still have to deal with the fall out.

November 18, 2006

My weight was down by 7.5 pounds. The half pounds counted for me when I was losing weight, but when I was gaining they were more of a rounding error. With 29 more to go, I set my focus on dropping 10 by Christmas. Once I did that, I'd drop another 10 before my next reconstructive surgery. That way, Dr. Sanders could suck the rest out with liposuction and I'd be back in shape by mid-2007, but I wasn't kidding anyone, not even myself. All of my planning was absolutely laughable. It was really more of a way to occupy my mind when I was alone because it seemed to have become crystal clear that I had no control over what was happening to my body. Instead of lying to myself about how much weight I could lose, I turned my attention to formulating outlines for a book that would tell my story. I asked myself questions like "If I didn't make it, what did I want my kids to know?" I couldn't imagine I would have the energy to write it in the first place, but if I did, how much detail could I share. Was it going to be a book for my family or a book for people like me? Would anyone even want to read it? There was no opportunity for me to further reflect on those questions because I lost that train of thought almost as quickly as it had pulled into the station.

November 22, 2006

Janet often drove me to my appointments in Madison, giving her an excellent opportunity to release some of the pain and hurt she had suffered in her life. I listened intently to her as she released a load of negative energy, then used a meditation clearing technique to force it out through a series of deep breaths. When we arrived at the university clinics, she guided me first to Dr. Harrison's office where he examined his handy work before concluding that the wound was healing well. Satisfied, he sent us to Dr. Paulson, a radiation oncologist at the University whose clinic was on the bottom floor of the hospital. Janet and I took the elevator down and when the doors opened into the dreary, low light dead end, I felt nervous to step out. I couldn't believe somewhere so bleak was equipped to help me recover. While it wasn't entirely obvious which direction we were to go in, there was some meager signage next to a heavy steel door. We passed through it, hoping someone would appear to help us choose which hall to go down and were quietly pleased when a woman wearing a scarf on what I assumed was her bald head turned the corner. She didn't say a word as she passed but helped us none-the-less. We traced her steps to the corner and did the opposite of what she had done, which got us to another narrow sign fastened on the beige wall, looking something like a name plate on a desk. It read "Radiation" with an arrow pointing in the direction we were going. Down in the bowels of the university hospital, the radiation oncology department felt oppressive and imposed an immediate psychological shift deep in my being. I checked in at the front desk with my new nurse Peggy who greeted me warmly before leading me to one of the exam rooms. Inside, she invited me to sit and asked some random questions before walking out.

At the door, she turned and said, "The doctor will be in shortly. Are you comfortable?"

I nodded my head and Peggy shut the door behind her. That was around 12:15. About 30 minutes later, she returned to tell us Dr. Paulson was just finishing up with another patient and would be in shortly. When another 30 minutes had passed, a medical student stopped in to ask me a couple of irrelevant questions, turning my light bulb on. "Pop-ins," as I called them, were timed at 30-minute intervals, designed to diffuse the patient's building frustration just like being on hold with elevator music streaming through the earpiece. When Dr. Paulson finally did arrive, our exchange was short and sweet. He felt my throat, asked about my breast cancer and said Peggy would schedule an appointment for me to be measured for a full-face mold from which they would create a plastic mask for me to wear during radiation treatments. After scheduling my next appointment, Janet and I were finally released at 4:30 p.m. It was that way each time I had an appointment at the university hospital. No matter what time my appointment was, the entire day would be consumed in their oppressive and uninspiring academic halls.

November 27, 2006
The morning I was to have a mold made of my face, I was instructed not to eat after 9:30 a.m. Uncharacteristically, I ignored them and ate a clementine on the drive in. I can't tell you why or what I was thinking only that I felt oddly detached from that next round of cancer treatment. Maybe I was in denial about the seriousness of the mucoepidermoid carcinoma and was holding on to the initial assumptions that it was low-grade. Of course, it wasn't. It was high-grade, but I still couldn't find any reason to worry. I was either deeply depressed or doing really well with my meditation practice, which was guiding me towards a more peaceful existence. It was a horse apiece.

Dr. Paulson explained, "We have an excellent technology. It delivers radiation treatment to just the tumor and was developed right here in Madison. It's called Tomotherapy. The Tomotherapy machine delivers a tight 3-D dose of radiation around the affected tissue, sparing the surrounding areas and reducing your risk

156

of losing teeth while it minimizes the tissue damage around the tumor site. The mold we're creating today will be used to fashion a mask of your face and the front half of your head. During your treatments, you will lie on your back with the mask over your face and fastened to the table. That way you can't move your head and cause us to radiate the wrong area."

The only response I had was "OK." I had no questions, no concerns, just OK. While I waited for the technicians to take me in for measurements, I found myself lost in the tranquility of understanding that I was using everything God had provided me. I had a deep sense of knowing that there wasn't much more for me to do other than stay open to new things coming my way. I believed with all of my heart that God was nudging me down the path he had designed for me, and if I had described that feeling before I had actually felt it, I might've characterized it more as empowering, but it wasn't that at all. It was more like a peaceful knowing of something I couldn't quite put my finger on. The only explanation that resonated for me was that I was evolving, meaning moving closer to the person I was meant to be. Along the way I had danced around the idea of fully embracing integrative medicine, which tied together a variety of practices including massage therapy, meditation, mindfulness, acupuncture and reiki to promote my healing. The use of complementary medicine with conventional medicine had become known as integrative medicine, which meant working to heal the whole person. Using food as medicine and meditation to fight cancer was just the beginning for me. With Janet's help I dove deeper by adding reiki, also known as universal energy, to my toolbox.

At one of her art shows, Janet met a photographer by the name of David. David had recently completed his studies in reiki to become a master and was increasing his strength by working on friends and family. So when Janet approached him to work on me, a cancer patient, he was somewhat reluctant. He was just discovering what his true abilities were and wasn't sure what he could do for me but agreed to try. We met at Janet's cottage on the day following my third radiation treatment. He was nothing like what I had expected. Dressed in khakis and a navy-blue polo shirt, David's white hair gave his age away, but nothing about his outward appearance told the deeper story of his astonishing gifts. He began our session by explaining what he was attempting to do for me, and without any fanfare, he gently instructed me to lie on the massage table and relax. Ideally he hoped I would close my eyes and fall asleep, but if I wanted to keep my eyes open, that was fine with him as well. Admittedly, I was quite confused by what was about to happen, but honoring my commitment to stay open, I took in a deep breath, blew it out and closed my eyes.

As I relaxed on the table, I heard David take in three deep breaths and slowly release them from his lungs. I opened my eyes briefly and saw him with his hands together fingertips facing up in what I now know to be Gassho, the symbolic prayer position. He proceeded to "sweep" the air above my body, and feeling embarrassed to watch what seemed like an intimate act with his creator, I closed my eyes again. Moments later, he listed the areas in my body that were ailing. I hadn't given him any details except to say I was battling cancer, so I was dumbfounded as he named every physical challenge I had dealt with during my entire life. His hands hovered just above my clothed body, emanating a strong surge of heat that at times became almost unbearably hot. When he was done he swept the air above my body again, shook out the energy and went to the sink to wash his hands. I felt a little fuzzy as I stepped down from the table and dropped into a nearby chair.

"How was that for you?" David asked.

"I don't know. I'm not sure what THAT was," I responded.

"Today, I was working to clear your energy and balance your chakras so your body can begin to heal. I didn't want to do too much because I think it would've been too hard for you to physically handle today. So, I will do more next time. I can tell you that your breast area is clear and there are no further problems there. So, that's great news. Over the next 24 hours, you may experience soreness throughout your body and may also find yourself crying without reason. It's all part of the cleansing and releasing your body needs to do before the healing can begin. If you're open to it, I'd like to meet with you again because I think there's much more I can do for you."

"That would be wonderful. Thank you," I said without giving my answer any thought.

I wanted to believe him, but later, I over analyzed my time with David and struggled to understand how he could possibly know that much about me and do what he said he does.

December 8, 2006

The Carbone Cancer Center at the University of Wisconsin-Madison called to tell me they had switched my appointment times to the following week, and that was that. They weren't calling to see if the new times fit into my schedule, it was just expected that I would make the change. There was no apology or recognition that the change might inconvenience me at best or at worst throw me into an all-out anxiety attack. It was one of the most glaring differences between my hometown cancer center and the complexity of a university research facility. At home, the cancer center worked around my schedule, accommodated my kids and did everything possible to reduce my stress short of offering onsite childcare. At the university, there was no recognition of how difficult it was for parents to manage childcare through cancer treatment, and making those last minute changes inevitably made an already impossible situation much worse. Ironically, counseling during cancer treatment focused heavily around reducing stress but never discussed the burden of childcare. Had my cancer clinics offered childcare onsite, I could guarantee that my stress levels would have dropped exponentially. I'm sure the prevailing belief was that a cancer clinic was nowhere for kids to be, but my children and I were always happier when we were together. At that point in our lives, we all would've preferred for them to be with me drinking apple juice and eating graham crackers rather than being shuffled around from one person to the next. It was clear to all of us that I needed my kids as much as they needed me, and being separated from them so often and for so long was taxing on us all.

December 17, 2006

My health was weighing heaviest on EmmaGrace. One morning when Ron dropped her off at school, her teacher was waiting to talk with him.

"EmmaGrace just isn't herself lately. She flunked two tests and got a C- on another one, and I know she can do better. She's also uncharacteristically rude and mean to the other kids," Mrs. Walters reported.

"We'll talk to her after school," Ron said and waved good bye to EmmaGrace.

Later that day we asked EmmaGrace what was going on, but her only response was, "I don't know."

"Honey, you're never rude to the other kids. Something must be going on for you to act that way. Did something happen?" I asked giving her another opening.

"Two older boys told me you were going to die. I told them you weren't and they said you were because you had two cancers," EmmaGrace finally blurted out.

"Why didn't you tell us what happened," I asked.

"I didn't want to hurt your feelings," she responded looking down at the ground.

I explained, "My feelings can't be hurt by people who don't know what they're talking about. People say a lot of things out of their own ignorance or fear. It's important not to pay attention. Find compassion for them and recognize how hard their lives must be for them to be so negative and wrapped up in someone else's business."

The next day her teacher reported back that EmmaGrace had apologized and was back to her normal cheery self. Just like that.

With one week of Tomotherapy down, Monday morning greeted me with a new routine. I left the house at 7:50 a.m. for the one hour drive to Madison, parked in a massive parking garage and made my way down the many levels of concrete stairs masquerading as my daily exercise. The University of Wisconsin Carbone Cancer Center was a hard place to spend time. Each day, I found myself caught up in a stream of patients suffering with difficult maladies. Deeply saddened to be a part of that somber parade and hobbling in through the electronically revolving doors, I skirted around its edges failing to avoid eye contact. On that morning, I passed a mother guiding her downcast daughter, who obviously suffered from anorexia and was nearly too weak to walk on her own. I smiled weakly, meeting the mother's sorrow-filled eyes and held the manual door for an elderly woman whose gnarled arthritic hands and feet struggled to get her walker through the opening. Once inside, I tried to walk faster down the hall but was slowed by a man in a wheelchair, pushing himself along with his feet. He was too deformed to lift his head and look at me, even though he tried. I waved my hand down low so he could see me greet him and quickened my pace passing him. Finally in the radiation oncology waiting room, I paused before sitting down to watch the technicians lead a man with Down Syndrome into the Tomotherapy room for his treatment. While I felt detached from everyone I saw, it was undeniable that I was as much a part of their day as they were of mine. I reflected on how nice it would've been if we had been introduced as comrades in convalescence instead of cohorts in calamity.

I drove myself to Madison when I could and asked friends or family to drive when I was far too tired. On one of those days my sister signed up for what we decided would be a somewhat fun day with EmmaGrace. After my treatment, Karen took us to Bernie's Rock Shop. We were all rock hounds and joyously lost ourselves for hours picking through piles of stones. Another time Ron drove and we took the girls to Olbrich Gardens where a Thai Sala, or pavilion, was displayed, having been donated to the University of Wisconsin-Madison by the Thai Government. From the gardens we went on to the Madison Children's Museum where I sat and watched the girls discover how energy worked and applauded as they harvested wooden vegetables from a foam garden bed covered by a brown sheet. I found a modicum of joy in those field trips, which redirected the attention away from my wretched plight.

December 23, 2006
I was overwhelmed with the number of people poking and prodding me. The doctors and students at the university hospital were so interested in my case that I became a living classroom, playing host to droves of students filing through my exam room while I sat on display – the freak with two rare and aggressive cancers that may or may not be connected. "Look at her, she's still alive," I was sure I heard them say. I was the third patient and the only one living that Dr. Paulson had treated with IBC and mucoepidermoid carcinoma, and he believed there might be a link between the two. Early research showed a connection between both cancers to the chicken pox virus. Even so, I was done with strangers busting into my intimate space and finally got up the nerve to end it.

When the resident came into my room, handed me a gown and asked me to change, I stopped her before she could let it go and said, "I am here for head and neck cancer, not breast cancer. I'm not going to change into this gown anymore."

She smiled and said, "I wondered how long it would take you to call us out."

"I didn't know I could," I said.

December 26, 2006
My throat was always sore, my lips were puffy, my mouth and left cheek hurt, and my tongue was smooth. Apparently, my taste buds were gone, which explained why food tasted rotten again. Janet gave me calendula and comfrey salve for my skin and lips, which was purported to help the cells regenerate more quickly, but with 10 treatments down and 20 more to go, I clearly needed something more powerful. I called Reiki Master David who had continued his training since our first session and brought some new techniques to the table. Because of my extreme exhaustion, I had no trouble relaxing. My body went limp, melting into the table as he worked his energy healing magic. The left side of my head felt like it was being sucked into a vacuum hose, which was both intriguing and terrifying but didn't hurt. Even though David wasn't touching me, it felt like he was and it freaked me out so much that I kept my eyes closed tightly so I couldn't see what was happening. It was probably the opposite of what I should've done, but I trusted that he was doing what would ultimately help me, believing he was my last hope. When it was all over and I was off the table, David sat down with me to recount what had happened, which left me confused by what was real or imagined.

"How is your throat?" he asked.

I swallowed and realized it no longer hurt.

161

My eyes widened in disbelief as I answered, "It doesn't hurt."

David smiled and said, "It shouldn't hurt any more. Did you notice any other changes?"

I said, "Not really. It just felt so weird to have my head sucked into the shape of a cone like being sucked into a vacuum tube like I used to do on my skin when I was a kid. I was too afraid to open my eyes."

He laughed, "I wondered what that would feel like or if you would feel anything at all. I was pulling the excess radiation out of your head along with the negative energy it left behind." Then, he handed me a mirror and said, "Take a look at your neck."

I took the mirror and tilted my head to better see the radiated area. It was no longer red. I moved over to the window for better light and still couldn't see the red rash that had been there when I had walked in through the door. I looked at him in disbelief and David, my reiki master, let out a little giggle. It was at that exact moment, unbeknownst to me, that my personal transformation had begun.

December 29, 2006
With 14 treatments down and 16 more to go, I was having trouble turning my head because of the scar tissue forming at the parotidectomy site. Instead of appealing to the doctors for help, I went back to David, and after a 90-minute reiki session, my neck loosened up. The following day, Dr. Paulson examined me and was just as stunned by the elasticity in my neck as I was. In between reiki sessions, my mouth hurt and my stomach ached. My ear, neck and throat throbbed with a strong dull pain, and David suggested he work on me more often to help manage the accumulating side effects. I wished I could've, but I didn't want to be around people that much. I needed time off and that meant enduring pain. On top of it all, I got the respiratory flu, which was wildly inconvenient during my Tomotherapy sessions as I tried to breathe with my face pinned under the plastic mesh mask. Fantasies about being done with doctors, clinics, hospitals, tests and most importantly cancer filled my empty thoughts.

The peace I had felt at the beginning of the process had faded once again, and I found myself focusing on everything I hated. I hated the sound of the Tomotherapy machine. I hated the smell of the room. I hated the mask so much that I developed anxiety at the sight of it. I hated the way my technician, Eric, asked if I wanted a blanket. I said no every day, but he kept asking anyway. I guessed it was part of protocol, and there was no way for him to part from that sacred protocol. The moment I crossed the threshold into the scanning room, I developed nausea. A wave of vomit threatened to erupt each time I saw the masks lined up on the wall looking like ghostly images of other cancer patients. I considered mine and how I didn't want to end up just like it, sitting on a shelf somewhere in the bowels of a morgue. I worked so hard on meditating and visualizing myself calm, peaceful and healthy but was failing miserably. With 14 more treatments to endure, I thought I had to try harder.

January 5, 2007
I arrived at the UW-Madison Carbone Cancer Clinic once again for a long day of appointments, but when I got to the radiation department, I was informed that the machine was down. Why they hadn't called their patients in the morning when they knew the situation was beyond me. It was Friday and they expected me to return the following day but I looked forward to the weekends when no one would invade my personal space and couldn't stop the little howl ejected from my lips.

I cried in protest,"I'm thinking of quitting anyway," I told Eric. "They said they got the tumor with good margins and there wasn't any visible cancer in the tissue surrounding the tumor. I probably don't even need more radiation. So, I'm not going to come back tomorrow."

Eric's eyes widened. He moved to the phone, picked it up and spoke quietly into the mouth piece as if he was a ward at a psychiatric hospital. He had called Dr. Paulson and I overheard him tell him to come and manage his own patient. Seconds later, Dr. Paulson arrived by my side, took one look at me and announced a three-day reprieve. Then, he sat down to explain how the radiation worked on cancer.

"The reason we have you suffer through 30 treatments of radiation is because of the way cancer works. There may very well be cancer cells that we didn't see on the scans or in the margins of the tumor. We wouldn't want to have you back in a year's time. So with the first 17 treatments, the cancer cells are in shock and weakened. By the 27th treatment, they are all dead except for a handful of really tough ones. With the 30th treatment we know we've gotten them all. So, I need you to keep going and get to 30. If you quit now, the net effect is zero." he gently implored.

Then on a brighter note, he said, "You're handling the effects of radiation really well. Your neck should be much redder by now and your throat should be very sore, making it hard for you to swallow."

"I have a reiki master," I said without emotion.

163

He gave me a cockeyed look. I explained what David did and watched as the doctor accepted what he could see with his own eyes but might've denied in theory. Dr. Paulson was so taken with my results that he asked me to speak to a group of patients and healthcare practitioners about reiki. My first reaction to his request was that I was just too tired to do anything extra, but his encouragement lifted my spirits. I realized that by revealing my secret, I might also be able to help someone else, so I agreed and invited David to join me. That simple request by Dr. Paulson secured my resolve to finish what I had started, compelling me to show up for radiation the following Monday.

Several days later during my presentation to a group of patients and healthcare workers, I could see that the group was accepting reiki as an option for managing side effects. It was obvious to even the skeptics that it was working for me. In the hall afterwards, I asked Dr. Paulson about the patients in the room and where they were at in their treatment, noting how frail they appeared.

"Each one of those patients is more than one year out from their treatment. Some are two. You were the only one in the room still in treatment. The medical staff told me they couldn't believe how healthy you looked," Dr. Paulson said grinning ear to ear, exuding pride.

My example of using meditation, reiki and food as medicine happened before the University of Wisconsin – Madison Medical College had established their integrative medicine program, and I like to think that my case gave them a little support for what some were already contemplating. Today, their integrative medicine program helps patients work through health challenges in ways not yet defined by treatment protocols, but I believe it's only a matter of time before protocols catch up.

January 11, 2007

Each day I found myself speaking less and less out loud since there was more than enough conversation happening in my mind. My taste buds seemed to be overlooked by reiki and were so damaged that most foods tasted wretched. I once again restricted my diet to "non-offensive foods" including: rice, bread, eggs, artichoke dip, fruit smoothies, salads, hummus, oranges, lemon water, eggs, vanilla ice cream, and orange, cranberry, or grapefruit juice. I no longer ate meat because its flavorless texture felt like gritty paste in my mouth. I had no other choice but to choke down food. If I had stopped eating, my body would certainly weaken, leaving me vulnerable to a cancer recurrence. So I committed to doing what was necessary to win and forced down, eggs, fruit, and salad with a chaser of brown rice. I continued to be deeply motivated by the idea that my girls needed to see me as brave and strong. Imagining them as young women facing challenges of their own, I hoped they would draw strength from my example. Even though I no longer felt that my death was imminent, I still reflected on the possibility that EmmaGrace and Hannah would face a future without me, and if that happened, I wanted there to be no doubt that they could be as tough as I had been– no matter what.

As I moved through treatments, Dr. Paulson noticed that I was becoming more withdrawn and suggested, "We have a very skilled cancer psychologist named Dr. Markus. You might find it helpful to pay him a visit. Would you like us to set up an appointment for you?"

"I suppose," I agreed, still somewhat obedient to conventional wisdom even though I heard a small whisper of a suggestion deep in my soul that what I really needed was more meditation to usher in a metamorphosis of sorts.

On the third floor of the hospital I studied the moss green walls in Dr. Markus's 12' x 12' room. It was furnished with one leather recliner, one hard backed upholstered chair and one leather couch. Sitting next to the couch was a small side table on which a box of Kleenex sat with one sheet already drawn out and standing at attention in case I needed it. I sat upright in the recliner, leaning forward with my hands under my thighs, left leg bouncing as I studied the detail of the room. Mentally I walked through what I wanted to say, but when I rehearsed it out loud, I sounded off my rocker. My thoughts seemed completely out of the realm of understanding for almost everyone I knew, but then again, it might be easier to talk with someone who didn't know me at all. How was I going to explain the emotional upheaval I experienced when I believed I would die, and yet knew that I wouldn't. How was I going to explain that I spoke directly to God and heard him speak back? How was I going to characterize my conversations with God that led me to understand that I was his tool for something but had no comprehension of what it was. My meditation practice didn't produce the kind of clarity others seemed to be blessed with, which left me confused by the notion that I was going crazy and yet knowing I wasn't.

The door opened and a slight, partially bald, middle-aged man quietly walked through, smiling and maintaining eye contact as he moved to the hard-backed chair and slipped onto its seat, crossing his legs and positioning his notebook on his lap in one single motion.

"Hello! I'm so pleased to meet you. I understand you are going through some very challenging times and I'd like to help you through them if I can. Would you mind sharing where you're at in your treatment and how you and your family are getting through it?" Dr. Markus gently asked.

I took a breath and let it all hang out. On one level, I had hoped he would tell me that talking to God and "believing" he was talking back was a side effect of my medication, but he didn't. Instead Dr. Markus explained what it meant to be kind, supportive and compassionate towards myself. He didn't directly address the transformation I felt like I was going through but moved me closer to a more clear understanding. He handed me a pen and notepad then asked me to write down all of my needs without thinking about them.

"Just write anything that pops into your mind. Don't judge it because I most certainly won't. What would you like more of in your life?" He asked encouraging me to speak my truth.

I paused looking down at the paper, cognizant of Dr. Markus sitting quietly in his chair. If I was going to get anything out of that session, I needed to pretend he wasn't there. So I pictured myself sitting at home, writing in my journal then started my list. After 10 minutes had passed, he lightly asked me to read them back first to myself and then to him. My list included, rest – lots of rest – exercise, time with friends, fun with my kids, music, quiet time to write and meditate, adventures during which I could be physically comfortable, good health, an emotional connection with Ron, and an understanding of why I was still alive.

I read the list back and asked out loud, "Oh, is that all?"

Dr. Markus softly laughed and instructed, "carry that list with you and read it over whenever you have a quiet moment. Don't judge it, just reflect on it and next time we'll move to the second part of the exercise. It was very nice to meet you."

January 13, 2007
I reviewed my list and stopped at "lots of rest." I was so tired.

January 18, 2007
Same.

January 24, 2007
I woke up with what seemed like the stomach flu, otherwise known by my doctors as a confluence of side effects. Pushing back with energy healing was getting harder in the mindset of wallowing, so I acknowledged that being sick was just a part of their game and as long as I chose to play along I would have to endure. I turned my attention to the more tangible task of evaluating where I was with my friends. For me, battling cancer was like a watershed of fate that brought together so many incredible people to help me – save me really. Some old friends stuck around, jumping in to help where they could ,but most faded

from view. They were burdened by their own fears around cancer and only reappeared when I resurfaced socially in 2010. For the most part, it was new friends that shouldered the weight of supporting my fragile emotional state. Cancer wasn't like other diseases. It's life threatening nature could elicit unexpected reactions, and the key for me was to expect the unexpected or, better yet, expect nothing at all from the people in my life.

January 28, 2007

EmmaGrace's exuberant, creative and fast paced personality set her apart from the other students in her class, making her a target for teasing that quickly transitioned into bullying. Struggling to deal with her own emotions and need to be compassionate towards others, EmmaGrace broke down one day after I picked her up from school. She cried the entire drive home, leaving me powerless to help her, not that she wanted me to. She blamed me. My sickness and consequently weakened condition became the root of all her problems. As the weeks passed, her constant requests that I "do" for her, presumably to make up for "it all," were difficult for me to keep up with even though I tried desperately to store some daily energy for her after school. It was the same each and every day. As soon as I got Hannah settled, I'd sit down to help EmmaGrace with her homework only to have her stop trying, showing no empathy for my state of being – weak, tired and sick from treatment - which I understood was unbearably repetitive at best. How could I feel hurt? She was only eight years old. On top of parenting through cancer treatment, I was a first time parent to an eight-year old daughter. I was learning too but felt like I was failing miserably. Cancer treatment brought on so many insecurities that I was left to agonize over decisions that might normally have been easy and natural to make. For example, should I ask EmmaGrace to pick up her toys or do it for her? Should I expect her to eat the food on her plate or make something special just for her? Should I be there whenever she called or help her recognize that I had important things to do as well? I lamented my inability to not keep up with being the type of mother I wanted and needed to be while fighting cancer, but Dr. Markus set me straight at our next appointment.

"You are a good enough mom. You do not need to be perfect. Saying no is part of parenting, cancer or no cancer," he coached.

Through waves of breast and lymphedema pain, hot flashes and fatigue, I read the *Invitation* by Oriah. It reminded me that Emma Grace was a child, and while it was my first job to take care of my kids, I also needed to take care of myself. Her book inspired me to look at EmmaGrace's intentions differently and focus on her loving heart and depth of caring, which she displayed whenever she played with Hannah or attempted to make us eggs for breakfast. Hannah also worked to brighten my miserable existence with dances, pictures

167

and hugs. The compassion my girls had for me was obvious and I wanted to mirror that compassion back to them, but I first had to develop compassion for myself.

February 2007
When the radiation treatments ended, I was anxious to end my ordeal and jumped right into focusing on the long awaited "final" reconstructive surgery scheduled for February 12. While I was nervous about the resulting pain, I was excited to be done. I searched for the silver lining and found "perky boobs" at the edges of my dark cloud, which I half-heartedly proclaimed would make it all worthwhile. Would it really? No, I admitted to myself, it would not. Mercilessly, my mental preparations were delayed by another bacterial infection colonizing in my compromised microbiome. I coughed out radiation-flavored gunk throughout the day while developing a mild fever, sore throat and chest congestion. Compelled by Dr. Sanders to keep him apprised of my health leading up to the surgery date, I called to report my symptoms, which left him no choice but to postpone my surgery and prescribe another round of immune system destroying antibiotics. Although I felt better within a day, I worried that my body would reach a point when antibiotics would no longer do the trick and then challenged myself to find another silver lining.

Out of the blue, EmmaGrace walked over to me, gave me a big bear-hug proclaiming, "Mom, you're losing weight! I can wrap my arms all the way around you!"

Ah, there it was. My silver lining for the day. She was right. I had lost 13 pounds and was so happy somebody had noticed. Hope, on that front, had been restored. Once the infection was resolved, my surgery went smoothly. I spared myself the pain medication, opting to use reiki instead, which left my mind clear for contemplation and pondering the term I heard absolutely everywhere, "cancer survivor." As I've mentioned before, I didn't like it at all. It felt so passive. I was an active fighter, working hard to find additional ways to combat cancer. For me, it wasn't so much about survival as it was about facing fears and taking on my foe with full consciousness and intent. It was the cancer that was trying to survive, not me. I was the "Victor" not the "Victim." I was a warrior for sure and could accept that label. I was an advocate, a formidable adversary, an informed patient, a self-preservationist, a "confrontationist." I was a winner, even though my body suffered from terrible pain, the newest of which was from deep bruising on the left side of my face from the brow down to my jawline. My lips were burned, headaches were persistent and mouth sores popped up relentlessly. Everything I ate tasted like metallic vomit, but the doctors were pleased and repeated that my symptoms were much more mild than expected. Even so, I felt terrible. Sometimes the warrior in me just wanted to lay my weapons down, leave the battle field and go home.

In lieu of an answer for what could be done, I noticed that my doctors often minimized the symptoms I suffered from prescription drugs, which only added insult to injury. Did they hope by playing down their significance, I would adopt the notion that my side effects were no big deal, therefore, reducing their impact on my daily life? While I understood the concept of mind over matter, I struggled to make it happen. Anger popped up much more often again. I was angry that the very treatment I was taking to save my life was just as easily able to destroy it. Perhaps it was Medical Darwinism, leaving only the strong to survive. More likely, my doctors didn't even think about it, having developed an insensitivity towards seeing the same thing over and over throughout their career.

"Tell me your symptoms today," they would ask.

Then, after hearing the extent of my list, their response was either a quiet humph as they typed it into their computer or the classification of them all together by Dr. Haper's favorite term "mischief." His word choice felt dismissive of my suffering even though he didn't likely mean it to be. I was sure it was hard to practice compassion constantly, but for my sake, it was important that my doctors always did. I wanted them to re-pledge to do no harm and stop assaulting me with toxic bombs. I wanted all of my medical practitioners to bring compassion back and practice the art of medicine by casting a broader net out into my potential treatment options to hopefully capture my salvation.

March 2007
With the help of Janet, I pushed back and attempted to engage in life outside my illness. She and I took Hannah and EmmaGrace for what was to be my first "normal" night out in nearly 18 months. We planned to enjoy dinner followed by a play at the community theatre then home before 9:00 p.m. Regrettably, half-way through dinner Hannah threw up. The majority of it hit her plate, but as I scooped her into my arms and ran for the bathroom anticipating another round, the next bout exploded all over me. I nearly cried out to the whole restaurant, "All I want is a nice salad that someone made just for me! Then I want to sit in the play with my eyes closed and the kids engaged! Is that so much to ask?" Instead, I took the girls home, bathed Hannah, showered and went to bed.

Every day, the bones on my face pulsated with pain. It wasn't hard to imagine the radiation still hammering away at my tissue, going after rogue cells like the game Whac-A-Mole. Purple blotches showed up on my lips with my tongue growing more painful by the hour. On the bright side, my taste buds did seem to be returning and Dr. Paulson validated what I thought to be true by explaining how radiation overspray had hit my tongue. Since mouth wounds heal pretty quickly, my taste buds would be back in service before too long, renewing hope that this foodie would enjoy the flavor of food once again.

On the farm, spring was in the air and the thick blanket of snow was melting into puddles on the lawn. I could actually feel the trees, plants, grasses and animals let out a sigh just like I was doing. Wisconsin was always the same on that first warm and windy spring day, evaporating the snow and exposing patches of grass that beckoned us to emerge from inside our homes. Anxious to stretch our limbs after a frigid winter, we donned sweat shirts and ran for the green. As the landscape of our farm released a wellspring of new life, so too did the landscape of my mind and body. I stretched my thinking from living off our garden to living off our land, starting with the maple trees. I did some research into maple syrup and found that, among other things, it showed promise in reducing the risk of prostate cancer. I extrapolated that if that was possible, then it could also help me prevent a recurrence. We invested in a complete tapping kit to collect another food right out our back door. We had several large silver maples shading the yard, which were not the favored variety for syrup due to the lower sugar content in their sap, but I wasn't concerned about that. We called the biggest silver maple the *Giving Tree* after Shel Silverstein's book by the same name. It was already our favorite climbing tree and held swings suspended from its branches, so why wouldn't it want to give up some of its sweet goodness to keep cancer at bay?

We carried our simple equipment to the base of the tree and thanked it for being so generous before Ron set the tap. It was only a couple of seconds before a clear liquid, a little thicker than water, dripped from the spigot and made a loud plopping sound as it hit the bottom of our plastic bucket. We all cheered! I held a cup under the metal tap as our giving tree let loose and gave the girls a taste. When the bucket was full, we carefully poured the sticky sap through a large felt like filter into another bucket, which we then poured into a seven-gallon pot waiting on the stove. For several days, the odiferous sap boiled, evaporating water and concentrating the sugar until the chemical reaction finally turned the sap from a watery clear color to a rich viscous amber, reminding me of my favorite stories as a child. The *Little House On the Prairie* book series vividly described maple syrup season and its scenes were coming to life right before my eyes. I relished the ability to replicate them in our own small way.

I took stock of the other trees and shrubs scattered throughout the 60-acres we called home. We had black raspberry bushes, hickory, plum, apple, cherry, and elderberry trees, and a booming black walnut grove. We were moving closer to subsistence living, which gave me an even deeper sense of connection to the earth. I focused next on the black walnut trees, which were mostly known for their beautiful wood since the nut was too bitter to enjoy. I discovered that the lime scented green husk of the nut carried significant healing properties and while WebMD noted that more evidence was needed to rate the effectiveness of black walnut tincture, the website did recognize its beneficial use against leukemia, diphtheria, syphilis, intestinal worms, skin wounds and other conditions. I urgently revived my prayers for scientists, hoping they would get the research dollars they needed to adequately study black walnuts and other whole foods for their potential to heal. Perhaps then they would discover a way to prevent chronic disease with the use of food, or at the very least, they might find a way to add disease fighting foods to treatment protocols and be able to reduce the amount of toxic treatments causing some to die and others to suffer irreparable harm. I planned to take an inventory of the medicinal plants growing around our house, hoping to have a better shot at keeping my family healthy and recovering myself more quickly. I was exhilarated by the thought that if I could just learn how to use it, the pharmacy right out my back door could help me heal.

March also brought another birthday for me and the gift of a new chicken coop designed and built by Ron to house the chicks that would grow to give us clean, quality, pasture-raised chickens and farm fresh eggs. While I was nervous about the responsibility that came with taking care of more lives, I was also thrilled. Farm fresh eggs had a flavor like no other. When cracked open, the yolk was a beautiful deep orange color packed with nutrition unlike the pale-yellow yolk of the store-bought version. Both the eggs and chickens would be packed with anti-inflammatory Omega-3 fatty acids and free of chemicals and antibiotics. Unfortunately my enthusiasm for our expanded farm life was dampened once again by yet another infection in my left breast where a couple of stitches had poked out. Another round of antibiotics was ordered and administered on my 43rd birthday, and while my special day was relatively uneventful, it was another birthday and for that I was grateful.

Five days passed and the antibiotics weren't working, so a stronger version was added in the hopes that they would hit their mark. It was becoming very clear that during the preceding months, I had taken way too many depleting the good bacteria in my gut designed to keep me healthy while the offending bacteria grew stronger and more resistant to the drugs. With less good bacteria in my intestines, my immune system grew weak, arresting my recovery. Colleen at my pharmacy was concerned as well and asked me to add probiotics to my daily routine. Probiotics packed with good bacteria, would replenish my gut and play a huge role in strengthening my immune system. So, I included foods like yogurt, kefir and soft cheeses to my daily meal plan along with fermented foods like Kimchi and sauerkraut. I also ate more prebiotics, which provided a food source for the probiotic. Since I was already eating some prebiotic foods such as asparagus, legumes, honey, and maple syrup, I was able to build from there with Jerusalem artichokes, garlic and onions. Understanding my microbiome gave me yet another tool to further protect my depleted body against a cancer recurrence because even though I was still in treatment, recurrence was a real possibility.

My doctors kept me committed to Aromasin, but I absolutely hated it. Not only was it a daily reminder that cancer could still be lurking in my body, but it gave me severe headaches, body pain and left me in a general cloud of dread that I dragged around with me all day long. Even though I wanted to move on and forget about cancer, the medical world wasn't ready to let me go. The silver lining? At the time, I supposed it was better to take Aromasin than to die.

I struggled to find things to do with my girls that didn't drain the tiny bit of energy I woke up with, and that's when I discovered another silver lining, Walmart. It became my standard offering after dinner when Ron was working late. It was easier to entertain them there than at home, and I could use the cart like a walker as we moved through the aisles. Each trip had a theme based on our needs at home. For example, craft day, clothes day, household goods day or toy day. The girls had a great time filling the cart with what we needed and then pulling it all out again to place it on the conveyer belt at check out. The low prices caused me to think about who might be suffering so that we could buy cheaply, but I couldn't dwell there too long because I selfishly didn't want to lose the only "playground" time I had with my girls. It was embarrassing to say, but I ignored my conscience.

April 2007
In the early part of April, I woke up with the bottom left quarter of my face achy and swollen. I noticed pain in my right arm and had a moment of panic before I realized it was lymphedema and not a heart attack. Depression was looming large and the infection in my left breast still had not acquiesced to the barrage of antibiotics. As hard as I worked at not focusing on what could be, the stress of knowing that cancer could rear its evil head at any moment crushed my entire being. To stave off despair, I refocused on my growing enthusiasm for our newly organized organic family farm. The large garden was ready to plant, the chickens would arrive in May and the cows were already growing healthy and strong in the pasture. For the most part, we had replaced processed sugar with honey from a local beekeeper, syrup from our trees, and our well water tested clean of pollutants. I walked a tightrope between falling into a chasm of anguish and soaring lightly with the overwhelming sense of joy and peace I had from knowing that I was doing everything I could to stay disease

free.

Living in joy and peace was challenged regularly by one complication after another delivered by the unrelenting cancer treatment. On one afternoon I displayed symptoms similar to those of a blood clot, forcing my mom to rush me to the emergency room where I was met by a young technician with a very wide grin. She whisked me into the stark CT scanning room for tests and very cheerily reported that she would need to inject me with contrast before taking "some pictures." Her smile reminded me a little of the Cheshire cat in *Alice and Wonderland*. Since it was 4:10 p.m., I suggested I run up to the cancer center to have them insert the needle for the IV fluids, adding that I had very difficult veins due to scarring from overuse. She smiled again and assured me she was good at her job.

I repeated a phrase my dad had often used, "If you can't get it the first time, you're not allowed to mine for my veins."

Maybe I shouldn't have said that because it seemed to throw her off. Her smile changed to something less confident as she continued on with her task. I knew I was in trouble, but I let her try anyway, and it did not go well. By the time I jumped off the table, it was 4:30 p.m. I had missed my window, and the cancer center was closed. I glowered at her, and without saying a word, she left the room. When she returned she reported that she would move me to the ultrasound room where one of the emergency doctors would insert the needle. (If you didn't know this already, never let a doctor insert a needle.) I dutifully shuffled across the hall and climbed onto the exam table as I heard them ask my mom to wait in the next room. Thank God they did.

The doctor came in and proudly announced, "No worries. I can get a needle in anywhere using ultrasound."

What he meant to say was that he was going to slather my arm with Lidocaine, so I wouldn't feel him digging around for a vein. I looked away as he started his mining operation and from the corner of my eye tried not to notice the sanguine oxygenated blood spraying from my arm onto my clothes, the gurney and the floor. In the middle of my blood bath, the doctor eventually did find a vein and the result of my scan was significant blood loss, but no blood clots, which was noteworthy. In the end, the diagnosis was lymphedema in my head, neck and arm.

When I saw Dr. Paulson and Dr. Harrison at my next appointment and questioned them about the lymphedema in my head and neck, they admitted to not having wanted to alarm me with the expectation because they believed it would've come much later in my healing process. They ASS-U-MED they had more time to cover potential complications and left me hanging. Too bad. I could have been working with a physical therapist to minimize the fluid buildup and probably wouldn't have had a panic, not to mention a whopper of an emergency room bill. Trying to earn his money, Dr. Paulson emphasized that over the past 18 months I had been through more than most people had in a lifetime. I knew he was trying to validate my frustration in hopes that I wouldn't find my way back into depression, but he wasn't helping. He continued trying to flatter me by complementing me on how strong I was and how I had gotten through chemotherapy, surgery and radiation beautifully, blah, blah, blah. Dr. Harper had taught me that I didn't have to look far to find someone worse off, and while it was true, his words merely served to minimized my own experience. In my world, I was the one worse off, and according to Dr. Markus, it was just fine for me to be depressed, want to be alone and be angry because my cancer treatment was brutal, and it pushed my physical, mental, and emotional state to the brink. As I worked to keep moving forward on the medical, practical and spiritual parts of my evolution, I found it nearly impossible to keep my body, mind and spirit working in unison.

My feelings were often conflicted. When I thought about dying, I felt strangely calm. Obviously, it would happen to everyone at some point and no one knew how or when, but I was acutely aware that I could be dead within a year, and maybe it wouldn't be because of cancer. Suzannah worked with a doctor at Memorial Sloan-Kettering who had been cured of breast cancer only to step off the curb in front of her clinic and be killed by a bus. Anyone at any time could die. Was death so bad? I knew several people who had died and their loved ones went on. Hard as I tried, I couldn't find any sense of fear around dying. Healing occurs, lives reorganize and everyone continues to move forward. I worked hard to make the best of the time I had left, trying to be loving and happy around my kids but regrettably the mental effects of Aromasin were extreme. I had no tolerance for kid antics and found taking my own time outs was crucial to the sanity of my girls. To that end, I haunted Marshalls and Kohl's, wandering aimlessly through the racks where I never saw anyone I knew, the bathrooms were just a few steps away, and no sales people tried to push me to buy anything. I felt invisible there, which I preferred over lying on the couch at home thinking about how hard everything was as I yelled at my kids.

The effects of radiation were once again mounting despite regular reiki sessions with David. My lips blistered, my tongue was raw, and my face was puffy from the lymphedema in my neck. I had headaches, fatigue, hearing loss and constant pain in my left ear. The scar tissue from the IBC radiation and surgeries was itchy, painful and set off muscle spasms throughout the day. My memory was significantly compromised, and I often apologized for my inability to move thoughts out into coherent sentences, which was generally met with a little snicker or a dismissive comment about how I was just aging like everyone else. I knew they meant it in the kindest way, but I also knew hearing about the side effects of cancer treatment made most people squirm, so it was easier for them to find a way to normalize it. Even so, I was comforted to know that others in my position also forgot words, couldn't finish sentences or move thoughts from their brain to their mouth and out into the world. It was what it was and that was all there was to it. I was suffering from chemo brain, so there.

To address the swelling in my arm and face, I went for my first lymphedema massage. I never could've comprehended how heavenly it would feel to have Mary, the massage therapist, work the lymph fluid up and out of my arm. As she did, a cool wave of relief washed through my hand, into my arm and up to my shoulder, forcing the pooling fluid to dissipate out through the rest of my body. The girls and I decided to call her "Mary, Mary, The Lymphedema Fairy" and appointments with her became both physically and mentally therapeutic. To help keep the fluids from pooling overnight, Mary ordered a custom-made head wrap, glove and sleeve from a company in Germany at a cost of $1,500. When it arrived in the mail, I laughed in disbelief at its size. It looked like a huge oven mitt for my face and hand. The arm sleeve was like the padding worn by the person being attacked during police dog training.

May 2007
Spring brought a host of events centered around raising money for breast cancer research. At my hospital, families and friends were encouraged to pull together teams in honor of cancer patients they knew. It was a perfect opportunity for my mother-in-law. She had been looking for ways to show how much she supported me and pulled together "My Team" including my daughters, nieces, sisters-in-law, sister and mom. Even though my mom had broken her foot a couple of weeks before, she insisted on participating and walked the whole way with a smile plastered on her face, serving as a testament to where my strength had come from. While the event was meant to have a celebratory mood, it felt oddly somber to me. At the start, I anticipated a marching band, but instead a man, one of the small percentage of men who contract breast cancer each year, appeared on stage. He gave a speech about how the cancer center employees were like his extended family and "they always had great room service." While I'm sure others felt inspired by his words, I felt very uneasy. I couldn't possibly think of my medical team as my extended family even though I liked them very much, and unlike the speaker, I was looking forward to never seeing them again.

I spent my time on the walk contemplating how I could share what I was learning about using food as medicine together with energy healing to help other people beat cancer. I envisioned my hospital hosting an integrative medical program that provided patients with an organic box garden and chicken coop to use as a classroom where I could teach patients about food as medicine, invite chefs in to teach cooking methods that preserved the highest nutritional value of those foods and provide continuing education on current research. I wanted to know how we could minimize the long-term negative impact of cancer treatment. I knew we could do better, and I was more certain than ever that if I continued to live, I would use my own "program" as a model.

July 2007

Still on the downswing as the summer heat rose and tensions in our house grew, it was a tough month for Emma Grace who regularly unloaded her burden of uncertainty on me. It seemed she had entered a detoxifying process of sorts to rid herself of the emotional load levied on her by an endlessly sick mother. Her anger, frustration, fear and sadness spilled out all over, leaving me to tearfully conclude that my illness was causing her more stress than she could shoulder. I tried the words my therapist gave me like, 'it must be so hard" and "I'm so sorry," but those well-rehearsed phrases fell flat. So I offered to enroll her in CLIMB, a program for children who had a family member sick with cancer, and I somewhat urgently described it to her as the sort of club she and Hannah could do crafts at but would only have to talk if they wanted to. The "craft" part peaked her interest and I wasted no time signing her up.

My growing burden came in multiple forms, hitting me mentally, emotionally and physically. It seemed I couldn't go even one month without something cropping up and July was no exception. Along with a growing pain in my neck, I was losing strength in my hands. While I didn't feel it was urgent, I did believe it was noteworthy, so I called Dr. Harper who wasted no time getting me in to see a neurologic oncologist. Dr. Kurtis rushed me through yet another MRI to thoroughly scan my spine. Once the scans were processed, he came into the exam room carrying a manila folder full of black and white plastic films.

"Hello," he greeted me with a Swedish accent as he pulled out one film after another and firmly jammed them under the metal lip at the top of a wall-mounted back lit box.

Illuminated on the screen was every vertebra in my spine. I was fascinated by the pictures and studied them, trying to identify the problem as if I knew what to look for.

"So if you look here, you'll see two holes in your spinal cord filled with fluid," Dr. Kurtis said pointing out an area on the slide.

Like working on a page out of a *WHERE'S WALDO* book, I strained to find what he was talking about.

"I don't see what you're pointing at," I confessed.

"There, right here," he said motioning a circle around an area that seemed to show a tiny break in my spinal cord. "These are called syrinx and I believe them to be the culprit of the pain and weakness in your hand. However, you also have spina bifida, spondylosis, an extra vertebra in your pelvis, and arthritis throughout your spine. Have you ever been told about those conditions?" he asked.

Wide-eyed at the long list of "defects" in my spine, I quietly answered, "No. Only the arthritis."

"Well, the good news is that despite the plethora of things wrong with your spine, it is not hosting cancer," Dr. Kurtis said almost joyfully. "Now, to address the syrinx. We can install a syringoperitoneal shunt into your spinal column to drain its fluid into your abdominal cavity. However, as with any medical procedure there are risks."

He paused, allowing me time to digest what he had just said. It wasn't hard to read between the lines. Installing a shunt into my spinal column was risky business, but not doing it meant the syrinx could get larger and cause me to become paralyzed. I didn't know how I felt about either option and closed my eyes, taking in three deep breaths before they popped open with a third idea.

"What if I tried reiki to see if it could help drain the syrinx?" I asked relieved that there might be another way. "What if I did reiki for some period-of-time and then we did another scan to see if it was working. Wouldn't that be an option?"

Dr. Kurtis stared at me and then at the films on the light box before saying, "If we did nothing for an eight-week period, I think you should be OK. But nothing is guaranteed when it comes to the body."

"I guess I'd rather try something I know won't hurt me before having a surgery that clearly could," I asserted feeling bolstered by my idea.

If he was being honest, I think Dr. Kurtis would say he was just as curious as I was about the limits of reiki, and since there was no tumor found, it seemed like a no brainer to give it a try. While David and I worked to energetically heal the syrinx, my symptoms disappeared, and the follow-up scan confirmed that reiki was working. The syrinx did shrink, which meant I was no longer a candidate for surgery.

I celebrated my little victory only briefly before another physical exam with Dr. Harper highlighted two bumps and a rash along the incision line on my right breast. It looked just like the skin mets or caner recurrence depicted on the internet, leaving me no choice but to undergo another biopsy. Luckily, it turned out to be a weird patch of dermatitis caused by the radiation. I welcomed another bullet dodged and relied more heavily on reiki, calling on David to teach me how to help myself. I ordered the reiki CD he had suggested and got to work while also keeping my appointments with the Naparstek CDs. The amount of time I spent on reiki, meditation and visualization mushroomed into several hours every day. The pea green couch that once symbolized my ailing body was transforming along with me into my place of healing.

August 2007
Follow-up appointments continued and Ron drove me to see Dr. Harrison in Madison to make sure there were no signs of head and neck cancer recurrence.

Wearing a circular mirror on his forehead, Dr. Harrison scrutinized my face and neck closely before happily reporting, "I can usually see in a person's face if they are still sick, but you look very healthy. But so as not to appear too cocky, how about we confirm what I see with an MRI in November just to be responsible."

It was excellent news and on the way home, Ron cried, which caused me to break down. Through my tears, I called my mom to give her the good news and heard her crying on the other end with my dad. After I hung up with them, I called my sister Karen who joined the tear fest.

When I was finally done with phone calls, I said to Ron laughing through my own waterworks, "Good thing we weren't all in the same room, we probably would've drowned!"

I left a message for my brother, Ron called his mom and dad, and with all the important calls out of the way, I turned my attention to the potential timeline for recurrence. If the head and neck cancer was to rear its ugly head again, it would likely be within 18 months of my surgery, which was the same amount of time IBC was likely to recur from the start of chemotherapy. Since the IBC deadline had come and gone, I had a sense of victory over one beast and expected to do the same with the second. Embracing the notion that I was likely to be alive the following year, I allowed myself to revel in the joy of our healing garden. Even though fall was in the air, I wasn't ready to say good-bye to the wonderful produce still popping up and decided to plant another round of peas in the hopes that the temperatures would stay warm long enough for them to fruit. There was more than enough spinach and I was thrilled to see the cabbage heads finally growing. I looked forward to picking the wild grapes laced through the trees along our trails and the various berries growing wild in the prairie. If I spent enough time learning how to make jam and "putting up" the produce, I could almost feed our family entirely from the land we lived on. In healing me we were also healing the land after decades of abuse from "strip" farming and chemical applications to grow genetically modified corn and soybeans.

September 2007
The start of the school year meant I had little time for anything other than healing and parenting, which made it hard to believe I could have ever had time for cancer. I took time out for the Internet as I surfed for updated information on the two cancers that had taken up residence in my body, but there was very little new. Both were rare, which meant with so few people suffering from them, very little research money had been dedicated to their study. Funding sources primarily liked the big hitters, the ones making the most noise, if you will. In other words, decisions to fund particular drugs were likely based on which ones had the biggest demand, and therefore, could make the most money. The mucoepidermoid carcinoma in my parotid gland represented between 3-5% of all head and neck cancers, with head and neck cancers accounting for only 3% of all cancers. As such, information on survival rates was difficult to pinpoint. It's possible that my survival rate was as high as 55% after five years and 75% after 15 years, which was markedly better than IBC, but the few studies out there were unclear.

Being one of the most aggressive forms of breast cancer, IBC was affecting more than 30,000 women each year but was only about one percent of the total number of breast cancers diagnosed. In 2005, there was a survival rate of 48% after five years. Meaning 48 women out of 100 would still be alive after five years. Another way to look at it was that we would lose more than 15,000 women to IBC in a five-year period. After 10 years, there was only a 24% survival rate, meaning less than 7,200 women would still be alive. I couldn't comprehend making a decision to not research a cancer that was killing more than 76% of its victims. By 2015, the statistics were better, relatively speaking. Since MD Anderson in Texas established the first Inflammatory Breast Cancer Clinic in 2006, survival rates grew to approximately 65% after five years and 35% after 10 years. Hope springs eternal.

October 2007
Two days after Hannah's fourth birthday, Dr. Harper reported to me, "As far as

it is medically possible to know, you are cancer free."

The tears welled up in my eyes. I had a sense deep in my core that I was healed, but I found it hard to believe.

"How can you be so certain so early in my recovery?" I asked.

"I just have a feeling. Can I give you a hug?" He compassionately asked.

"Of course," I said.

After he left the room, I sat in my chair and wept. I was glad I was alone because it turned into my moment to celebrate the strength I had summoned with God's help. That room meant so many different things to me, and none of them were good. The nausea, dread, solitude, and the whole 'muster it up and smile to let everyone see how brave you are because then maybe you'll believe it too,' not to mention the 'staying positive is the best way to beat cancer.' My time there had been horrible, but then how could it have been? Medical protocols took me to rock bottom like an addict, stripping me of everything I knew and then inadvertently cleared the way for me to find a deeper way of healing, using food, prayer, meditation, reiki, and intentional living to secure my place among the living.

While Dr. Harper believed I was cancer free, he was like any other doctor who rightfully wanted to see it in black and white. So when he returned to the room, he had a printed list of orders, which included a PET scan, chest x-ray, bone density test, mammogram and bloodwork, stating that if they all checked out, I'd be "good to go" for six months before doing it all over again. Because no matter how certain my doctor's felt, they too held a nagging doubt that it wasn't possible for me to be fine.

I submitted to the battery of tests unable to trust what my soul already knew and found I was buoyed by their conclusion that I was in remission. A huge burden was momentarily lifted from my shoulders but not my heart. Too many people I knew in treatment were not getting the same news. Survivor's guilt was knocking at my door, which led me to more energy work and time in my garden, which provided a constant source of strength and joy. The squash, zucchini, tomatoes, carrots, cauliflower, beans, lettuce, turnips, broccoli and even some onions came up anew. We had so much food that canning became all-consuming for an entire week, and when it was all said and done, we were fully stocked for the winter.

Life challenged me time and time again as if testing to see how strong I really was. The beginning of October was uncharacteristically hot, and the effect of the heat on me was compounded by Aromasin, which made me dizzy, causing me to lose my balance and break my elbow on one day and sprain my ankle on another. Heaven forbid I should go any length of time without some physical crisis. Ridiculous! On one of those days I was having a wonderful time outside with my girls, when somehow I twisted my ankle walking on a flat surface. I had tennis shoes on and don't exactly know what happened except that I felt dizzy. Within that same week, my body uncontrollably crumbled in the heat, crashing face down in the dirt. Aware that I was prostrate, I tried to open my eyes, but all I saw was blackness. I made an attempt to lift my head and flip onto my back, but nothing happened. My left arm was stuck under my body and would not move. Then from out of nowhere, 9-year old Emma Grace emerged as my first responder. With the strength of an adult, she picked me up and rolled me on to my back as she slid an outdoor pillow under my head. Noticing that I winced when she moved my left arm, she grabbed another pillow from a nearby chair and placed it under my arm.

Then taking a step back, she asked, 'What else can I do?"

"I took a breath in and pushed out the words, "Call Dad and Grandma."

"Do you want Tylenol?" she asked somewhat urgently. "For the pain?"

"Just go ahead and make the calls," I answered.

For more than 30 minutes, the girls sat on the ground next to me waiting for Ron to get home. My mom arrived just after him and offered to stay with the girls while Ron took me to the hospital, but EmmaGrace was having none of it.

"I'm going with you to be sure the doctors do the right thing," she asserted.

We left Hannah with my mom, and Ron and EmmaGrace escorted me to the all too familiar ER. I must've looked pretty bad because they wasted no time taking x-rays and assessing the damage. The radiologist on duty reported I had broken my elbow. It was so badly broken that they were only able to stabilize the arm before sending me to a specialist who happened to be my brother-in-law. At that point, EmmaGrace decided to bow out, trusting that her Uncle Matt had the right credentials to be my orthopedic surgeon, and after viewing my films and examining my arm, Matt's verdict was decisive. His partner would reattach the broken piece of bone back where it belonged and I'd be good to go. As hard as I tried to employ the peace and calm I was learning through meditation, I lost it. I cried so hard, blubbering on about how I just didn't know how much more I could take.

181

"I want to crawl in a hole. I can't handle all of my issues. I am one disaster after another. I've had knee surgeries, blood clots, difficult pregnancies, abdominal adhesions, syrinx, arthritis, cancer - two times - multiple sprained ankles and now a broken elbow? For crying out loud when will it all be enough?" I asked.

Sitting across from me in his white lab coat and blue Crocs, Matt compassionately explained, "Surgery is a quick fix. It really will be relatively easy and you'll be sent home that same day. No overnight in the hospital required. On top of that, you can use your arm right away as well."

There was obviously no way for me to employ my body's natural healing abilities to realign my bone, so I succumbed to yet another surgery. The after effects of anesthesia lingered longer than expected, forcing me to fight harder against depression as I lived just around its edges. I pushed back at the "new normal" working to make being infirm my new reality. If I was going to remain among the living, I had to find a way to enjoy life in spite of it. Just as I had settled into yet another revised mindset, our little family was hit with more. Later that month, EmmaGrace was at the fence with a close family friend watching the steer graze when he lifted his head and unexpectedly charged the fence. Emma Grace's flight mode took over, and in a panic she turned to run and slammed right into the massive pine tree just a few feet behind her. There was blood everywhere, and we found ourselves back in the ER where her head took five stitches and her mouth took one.

Our mole hills grew into mountains when we lost our sweet boy, Albert. The story goes that our neighbors wanted to hunt on our land, but we wouldn't allow it. So instead of respecting our landowner's rights and hunting on the hundreds of acres they collectively owned adjacent to ours, the "neighbors" decided to poach on the little 60-acre parcel we had developed into a sort of wildlife sanctuary. To succeed, they decided to take out the only real threat to their operation – our dogs. They poisoned them by hiding a dish of sweet tasting anti-freeze in the tall grass adjacent to our house, knowing we would never see it. Accidental anti-freeze poisoning kills 1000's of dogs every year, but the actual number of intentional poisonings is mostly unknown. A dog doesn't need to lap up very much to die and the poachers knew it. Albert was the first to pass, and his death made me feel numb. We had friends over the following day and Katelyn, a psychologist, took note of how strangely apathetic I seemed, calling me out in an effort to keep me from diving back into the depths of depression.

I explained, "I've had a monsoon of disasters and I'm just too exhausted to cry. I feel so beaten down and struggle to register even the slightest emotions."

"While I realize I can't know how you feel, I can say that empathy and depression are not options over the long run," she said compassionately.

I rallied my emotional self, and only a week later I found my other dog Kie foaming at the mouth. I rushed her to the emergency veterinary clinic, and after a series of tests, they concluded that she would not survive the anti-freeze poisoning and needed to be put down.

"Honestly, I don't even know how she's still alive. Her numbers are off the charts," the vet reported.

"Well, I can tell you I heard something similar when I was diagnosed with cancer and I'm still here, so I'm not ready to give up on her," I pushed back with conviction.

"The kindest thing to do would be to put her down, so she doesn't have to suffer any more," he recommended somewhat argumentatively.

Irritated by his attitude, I asked for a few minutes alone with Kie and called David.

"David, what do I do? I can't lose Kie too," I pleaded.

"You're not going to lose her right now. Let's work together. I want you to turn the lights off and sit on the floor with her. After all the work we've done together, you have plenty of reiki in you to share. I want you to sit quietly with your hands on Kie's heart and stomach area. Then focus everything you have on sending healing energy to her body, and I'll be doing the same from home."

At first, I felt a little embarrassed, but it only took a couple of minutes before I felt something happening. I shifted my body position and leaned into Kie who was still in my hands. I can't explain what was happening, but I knew David and I were helping her together. After 15 minutes, I called the doctors back and asked them to put her on dialysis. Where that came from was a mystery to me, but they reluctantly agreed, explaining that it would be expensive and the outcome was likely to be the same. I agreed to take the financial risk and left Kie in their capable but skeptical hands, returning five days later to take her happy little self home.

While I signed out at the front desk and paid my bill, the vet approached me with a full-face smile and proclaimed, "Your dog is an absolute miracle."

November 2007

With Kie recovered, I focused on appreciating what we had created on the farm. Each day, the chickens were producing 22 eggs with rich dark orange yolks. Orange was the color we were looking for. It was evidence that their disease fighting properties were intact. Factory raised chickens lacked that same nutrient value, had a pale-yellow yolk and were high in the inflammatory inducing Omega-6 fatty acid that promoted inflammation. Eggs from chickens who were allowed to graze were not only more nutritious but were high in Omega-3 fatty acids, which carried anti-inflammatory properties as well. Furthermore, our eggs were provided by happy chickens, grazing on clean pastures, and eating grasses and bugs as they were meant to. I greedily ate our chicken eggs, embracing every bite as I beat back any disease still present in my body.

By mid-month, Timmy The Cow, as the girls dubbed him, was gone. I was repentant over his fate. When Ron had summoned the butcher to "take care of Timmy," I watched from the house window as he fed Timmy a pan of oats, but when he took his rifle out of the back of his truck, I moved away from the window. Timmy never even saw his grim reaper aim the rifle and pull the trigger, sending a bullet right between his eyes. As soon as I heard the shot, I cried, thanking the cow for feeding us. His strong body was hoisted onto the trailer and taken away for processing. In a couple of months, he would come back to us in little white packages that I would respectfully organize in our chest freezer. I knew Barbara Kingsolver would have consoled my guilty mind by saying, 'he lived a good cow's life' because Timmy had grazed freely on rich organic pasture and provided us with healthy red meat in exchange.

With zeal, I studied everything we put in our mouths and evaluated how it prevented cancer from ever darkening our doorstep again. Recently, I've read reports of studies discouraging the consumption of red meat. While I don't prefer red meat, I'd argue that the recommendation does not take into account animals raised in a natural, healthy environment, eating what they were intended to eat, and grazing on pastureland free from chemicals. If you're a red meat lover, that's what you're looking for. In fact, I believe if all our food was grown truly organically, skyrocketing rates of disease would drop dramatically.

December 2007

The constant tussle with depressive emotions continued to put a damper on my meditative and reiki practice. They were always the first activities to take a hit when I was preoccupied. It was a real mistake on my part. Had I stuck with my practices, I would have handled the challenges being thrown in my path much more gracefully. At an appointment with our family practice doctor, I answered a battery of questions, leaving her to conclude that I was without a doubt in full blown depression. In an attempt to resolve the "issue," Dr. Langstrom encouraged me to try antidepressants for a few months, and I fell for it, hoping a pill could speed me to recovery. Apparently, I had forgotten the lessons I had already learned about the impact of prescription drugs on my body and was brutally reminded over the following days. I felt more than terrible and called her to report that I was having even more bad days than before.

"I don't want to run the risk of missing even one good day because of how a drug makes me feel. So, I want to stop taking them," I pleaded as if she was shoving them down my throat.

"Sometimes, one medication doesn't have the same effect as another. I'd like you to try Effexor and see how you do on that. In order for you to really know how you feel on it, you'll need to take it for a few weeks and then decide. I'll send a prescription over to Tobins," Dr. Langstrom said without asking my opinion.

Only a few days had passed after starting Effexor when I realized it was messing with my ability to think. On it, I had a strange sense of floating with no ability to focus, but out of the blue I was reminded to be my own best advocate, so I called Dr. Langstrom again.

I made it clear under no uncertain terms, "Those drugs are just not for me. I'm not going to take them anymore and waste my days feeling more detached than I did without them.

Dr. Langstrom asked, "Can I pray with you?"

"No. I come to you for your medical skills not religion," I tersely responded.

I called the clinic to switch my doctor to Dr. Fickle and never looked back.

Later in the month, I asked some friends over for breakfast and a therapeutic walk on our freshly snow covered trails. During our walk, we noticed fresh footprints on the trail that led to a pool of frozen blood in the newly fallen snow. Our eyes followed the stain off the trail as it morphed into a blood smeared depression. Clearly, someone had shot an animal and dragged it from our property. Staring in disbelief at the crime scene in my peaceful prairie, I called the Dodge County Sheriff right where I stood, and in less than 30 minutes he arrived. He followed the drag track to the north side of our land where our neighbor had built a deer stand. He climbed up the ladder and found a bullet shell that fit the ammunition used to hunt coyote.

"Look. I'm going to be honest with you. You're going to catch this guy long before I could. If we do catch him, you can press charges against him for trespassing, which is a felony offense. A word of caution though, be prepared for the fall out," the officer advised with concern.

While I knew which group of hunters the poacher would've come from, I didn't know exactly who it was, but the mystery didn't last long. One week later while sipping coffee on the eve of Christmas eve, Ron and I noticed a truck driving back and forth on the road in front of our house, which meant the poachers were at it again. Ron went to the deer stand where the bullet shell had been found to see if anyone was there. When he arrived, a teenage boy greeted him from inside the stand.

Ron greeted him back and asked, "are you seeing anything today?"

"No. Not yet," the boy answered.

"Was that you who made that excellent shot last week and got a coyote?" Ron pried further giving the impression that he was impressed.

Proudly, the boy revealed, "No! That was my dad. He shot it right through the heart. He's really a good shot!"

Ron called me from his cell phone as he walked back to the house and I called the sheriff while he was enroute to the women's shelter with a car load of Christmas toys. I reported what Ron and learned and the sheriff changed his trajectory, arriving at our farm within minutes.

When he got out of the car he said, "I knew you'd catch him before I did. I noticed a group of hunters down the road. What would you like me to do?"

"I want you to arrest them for trespassing," I told him.

"You know that could stir up a whole can of worms," he said warning me of the potential repercussions.

"The can of worms was already stirred up, remember? They are bullies and a bully can only bully if you allow him to. I'm done allowing it," I said with impudence.

In that moment, I had realized I had been passively accepting their abuse, but my good nature had reached its end. The sheriff gave me a nod and got back in his car. No more than 10 minutes later, he drove up the driveway again followed

186

by a green truck. The sheriff got out of his car first and reported that the man who shot the coyote wanted to speak with me.

"Are you okay with talking to him? It was your neighbor, Dale," the officer asked respectfully.

"Sure," I responded.

After the Sheriff waved him out, Dale jumped down from the driver's seat and approached me with a confident swagger accessorized with a huge grin then said, "Hey, Kathy. You know me. Our kids go to school together."

I said, "Yes, that's right."

He said, "You don't want to press charges against me."

I said, "That's where you're wrong."

He said, "We're neighbors. Why would you press charges?"

I said, "We're neighbors. Why would you trespass and poach, not to mention kill my dog?"

I told the sheriff that they could leave. He sent them on their way and wrote up the paperwork for me to sign, letting me know the district attorney would be in touch, then wished us a Merry Christmas before resuming his toy delivery. About 15 minutes later the Fire Chief dressed in his Sunday best, appeared at our front door. He had been with the group in my driveway and wanted us to know that he had no idea Albert had been killed, and if he had, he would not be hunting with them. I was certain I didn't believe him when he apologized profusely, but I thanked him anyway, knowing he was just trying to save face.

Weeks later, the district attorney called to tell me that I did not need to appear in court because Dale had been caught in a number of lies and eventually admitted to trespassing and killing the coyote. He pled guilty to poaching and got a reduced fine but was charged with a felony and would not be able to carry a gun for some number of years. Even though his prosecution didn't bring my dog back, at least the message had been sent that I would stand up to the bullies and ultimately end their reign, or so I thought. Over the next month, that same group of degenerate hunters showed up often on the road in front of our house, forcing me to adopt a new tact. Once they parked their caravan of pick-up trucks, I drove my black suburban to where they were and parked just across the street. Obviously they knew I was there because we were the only cars on that relatively narrow desolate stretch of country road, but my safety never even occurred to me. I attributed that to my compromised mental capacity. I rolled down the window and lined my camera up to record who was there. The first time I did it, they stood by their trucks and laughed.

The next time I found them in front of our house, I rolled my window down to take more pictures when one of them asked, "What good will those do?"

I said, "I will have proof of who was here, if any of you cause me trouble again."

Another hunter said, "Don't you have anything better to do?"

I responded, "Nope. I'm just sitting around recovering from cancer. I've got nothing better to do than to watch you guys and take your picture."

They looked surprised by my frankness, looking down at the pavement apparently feeling shamed, they got back in their trucks and drove away. It was the last time I saw them in front of our house.

A couple days later, David came over for another reiki session since I felt too drained to do anything for myself and admittedly had become somewhat dependent on the feeling of peace that washed over me each time I climbed up on his table. I closed my eyes and let the tension in my body melt away. My body felt like liquid as it sank deep into the table. The peaceful darkness of the hidden reaches of my soul were lit by an explosion of white bursting into the "field of vision" just behind my closed eyes, sending a cool wave of tranquility to buoy every healthy cell in my body. As the light slipped away from my mind's eye, I was left with the distinct understanding that I had been cleared of the negativity that had overshadowed me the previous two years and was ready for a new more meaningful year to begin.

January 2008
EmmaGrace must've sensed my shift and wanted to understand the mechanics of what my body was going through. I tried to be creative with the analogies I offered her.

I explained, "You know how when it's been dry and the plants are dying from lack of water, and then the rain finally comes and the plants perk up, but then the rain keeps coming, creating a flood? Rivers swell, plants are washed away. Animals and people get hurt or die, and houses are destroyed. Then the rain stops. The sun comes out and there's a giant mess to clean up. That's cancer treatment in my body. My body was dying from the cancer, and when I started chemo I got even sicker, but then again so did the cancer. The treatment kept coming just like the rain and flooded my body as it searched for more cancer cells. Unfortunately, just like when the flood waters recede, the chemotherapy left me with a big mess to clean up. So, this is my year to start the clean-up. I don't know how long it will take before I'm back to normal, but it will come. OK?"

EmmaGrace was silent, and I didn't ask if she understood what I was talking about because that explanation had drained me of what little energy I had. Instead, I leaned in to give her a hug.I felt both of our bodies relax into one another and could've stayed in that embrace all day if she hadn't wriggled away to play with Hannah, leaving me satisfied with that one seemingly successful parenting moment.

January found me in conflict between the peaceful notion that I was done with cancer and depression, which seemed to have a life all its own. I practiced being positive and strong but felt vulnerable and isolated. No one in my family had experienced what I had and therefore found it impossible to truly relate to my not quite developed new self. To be perfectly honest, I wasn't sure how to deal with who I was becoming either. It was clear that who I had always believed myself to be had changed, and cancer left me exposed in the barren landscape they still called my body. I was visibly and invisibly scarred and unwilling to leave the tranquility of my house.

Most days I sat broken, alone and still in my pajamas at mid-day. I sobbed while listening to a radio talk show, hoping to lose myself in their chatter, until one day my ears tuned in to a woman telling her story of clashing with chronic illness and the consequently excellent work she was doing even so. She was a doctor, a teacher, an organizer, an entrepreneur and a healer. Motivated to help so many more people than she ever could do in her office, Dr. Rachel Naomi Remen took to writing several books, and the one being reviewed that day was KITCHEN TABLE WISDOM. Immediately drawn in by her soft commanding voice and captivated by her powerful story, I found a glimmer of light in her words. The hardest hitting line she spoke was "Most of us are surviving our lives, and now we need to learn to live them." When the interview ended, I called Ron expressing my dire need to read her book and demanded he pick it up from the local bookstore on his way home from work. He was barely in the door when I snatched it out of his hand and ignoring everything else, began to read it voraciously.

The very next day, I reached the end and lingered on the last page. My hands held it firmly without any motion to place it on the table next to my chair. An epiphany of sorts was forming in my mind. I had been fighting so hard to live only to find myself spending each day surviving in a state of melancholy. I gazed at the cover, and needing more, I opened the book again and began to read the reference pages when a listing for a cancer retreat center jumped off the page. It was an organization Dr. Remen co-founded in Bolinas, California, a small coastal town perched on top of a cliff straddling the tectonic plates of the San Andreas Fault. The center was called Commonweal, and I instantly felt eager to go there. I called their office and a man by the name of Waz answered the phone with a melodious little trill in his voice. With his first word "Hello," I immediately felt protected in his warmth. He made me laugh for the first time in many, many months. Not because he said anything funny, but because his voice embodied happiness and laughter. Through the span of wires connecting our voices, he emanated pure joy as he soothed my anxious need to be just exactly where he was.

"I need to come and see you," I said desperately holding the tears back.

"Well, let's make that happen. Let's get you signed up for our next available session, which is in October. Now, I know that seems quite a ways off, but it will come quickly. I promise," Waz said giggling, and I didn't doubt him for one single second.

February 2008
One little epiphany after another rocked the boat of my philosophy on life, changing my ideas almost weekly. I had always believed my life was full before cancer, but as I lay on the pea green couch recovering a little bit more every day, I couldn't help but admit that I had mostly just survived my days. I accomplished laudable tasks, kept up with my responsibilities, planned for the future, but in the end, I mostly never lived in the moment. Ultimately, none of what I had done really mattered because it was all predicated on "Do, lest ye be viewed as lazy," a motto I had adopted early in life. Clearly it was time to change my mindset, and as the Dalai Lama had advised, "change your mindset, change the world." So, I threw my negative feelings out the window, hoping they wouldn't return like a boom-a-rang and hit me in the head, then set my mind on change.

I used the mindfulness skills I was developing to focus on living each day as it came. While I had originally learned to relax and surrender to treatments, it was time to surrender to life. During one of my meditations, a surprising revelation surfaced, which raised the possibility of no longer taking Aromasin. In the short time I had taken the drug, my weight had climbed to a new high, and the additional fat cells I carried generated hormones that could be used against me. Since I was already in menopause, those same fat cells picked up the slack in my hormone production. So it seemed reasonable to assume that the more fat I

190

had, the better my chances were for a recurrence, and while the primary role of Aromasin was to depress the production of adrenal gland hormones, it seemed counter intuitive to suppress one hormonal source while creating another. If I went off Aromasin, I would no longer suffer from head and body aches, I could lose weight, have fewer hot flashes, and be less irritable, fatigued, sleep deprived, and nauseous. What would I be missing? Confidence that cancer was being kept at bay? That just wasn't enough, so I decided to do a little secret experiment on myself and temporarily stopped taking Aromasin. In just three days I was blissfully sleeping through the night, but fearing the forewarned, I resumed taking it while logging my brief experience to be reconsidered at a future date.

It was time for another appointment with Dr. Harrison, and while I waited to be called, I found myself feeling compassion for the other patients waiting along with me and considered their circumstances. They were all older than I was and looked much sicker in comparison. There was the unshaven man in a wheelchair, holding a bottle of dried blood in his hands. He had a catheter that came out from under his shirt and attached to a clear bag filled with dark yellow urine. Occasionally, he glanced around the room in a disconnected way, showing no real interest in anything or anyone. A few chairs down from me was an obese man sitting in a large recliner. His shirt was partially untucked from his belted pants, and there was a dark stain of some sort just under its fourth white button. He sat with his eyes closed, groaning as he shifted unable to find a comfortable position. When the nurse came by, he opened his eyes to meet hers, then very quietly and politely asked for a soda. He glanced at me briefly and I met his eyes with a gentle smile, noticing that his mouth was visibly dry and unable to reciprocate. It wasn't a stretch to see myself in their shoes sometime in the future, so I closed my eyes and prayed for their recovery as vigorously as I prayed for my own.

In the exam room with Dr. Harrison, I asked, "Can you please check out this new lump behind my ear?"

While I didn't believe it was cancer, I was unsettled by not knowing just what it was. He gently moved his thumb and index finger around the ball, trying to slide it in different directions before naming it scar tissue and most definitely not a tumor.

Later in the week, my hometown doctors continued their search for what they considered to be the inevitable. It seemed difficult for them to accept that my new PET scan was clear, the chest x-ray was clean, and the MRI's of my neck, head, cervical, and thoracic spine were also free from cancer. Adding to their confusion was the lab which found nothing of concern in my bloodwork. It was absolutely perplexing to them that my blood chemistry was improving. The only results we waited on were those of my breast MRI, which my medical team seemed confident would tell the story of recurrence. From their experience, I shouldn't have been doing nearly as well as I was, but I embraced each test result as if it was a foregone conclusion and focused on recovering from the multitude of damaging side effects I had sustained.

Chasing down side effects became a preoccupation of mine. My hearing was at an all-time low, and Dr. Fredrick encouraged a hearing aid for my left ear that would allow me to hear when I wanted to and rest when I needed to by putting my good ear down on the pillow, leaving my deaf ear exposed. I was excited by the prospect, and while I tried on different hearing aids, my hearing was crystal clear until a crescendo of pain and pressure overwhelmed my face several minutes into the test. Because Dr. Harrison had found the tumor wrapped around one of my nerves during surgery, he had to remove it along with my parotid gland, leaving not only scarring but nerve damage which was compounded by the side effects of radiation. Dr. Fredrick concluded that the aid wasn't going to work but suggested that I try again somewhere down the road. I was disappointed but not devastated. It was another blow against feeling normal, but I was spared the big expense of hearing aids because my insurance company wouldn't even cover them. I was flabbergasted by that. I lost my hearing due to cancer treatment. Shouldn't correcting the damage be considered part of treatment? Those of us battling cancer go through enough without having to scratch our way back day by day. It had become a part-time job for me to navigate the obstacles levied against me by my insurance carrier in order to get my bills paid even though I religiously paid my monthly premium. If Congress wanted to reduce the cost of health care, perhaps outlawing the aversion insurance companies have towards paying legitimate bills, and putting a cap on the price of insurance, prescription medications and medical services would be a good place to start.

In the days following my hearing aid debacle, the breast MRI results were released.

Dr. Tousignant called and asked, "Are you OK?"

I said, "Sure, why?"

"Because of your breast MRI results," she answered.

"What about my results?" I asked

"You haven't heard? There's another tumor," she said sadly.

192

"What? No one called to tell me that and my scan was last week!" I said.

Before she called I was a winner and if the cancer came back, I would know what to do to beat it back again because I was walking in the light. However, soon after that call, my happy little illuminated demeanor crumbled. I found myself back in the darkness of the cancer roller coaster. One minute I was down, the next I was up before flipping around in circles trying to sort out whether or not I believed my health care providers had made a mistake. It wasn't long before I found out Radiologist Dr. Kerry had read my results and wrote up his report without ever looking at my history or calling my doctors. He didn't even send my results out until a week had passed, and then, he only sent them to my OBGYN.

"His report also says you refused an ultrasound or a mammogram. What does that mean?" she asked clearly baffled by his comment.

"I have no idea. He never even offered those tests to me. In fact, I never even saw him and this is the first I'm hearing the results. Was he trying to cover his fanny because he screwed up? Do doctors do that?" I fired a question back at Dr. Tousignant.

"None that I work with. I'm going to call Dr. Doering and see what he knows. I'll call you back," she said hanging up with a sense of urgency.

Several minutes later the phone rang and I snapped it up before the first ring ended.

"Hello?" I answered questioning if the caller was my doctor.

"It's Dr. Tousignant. I spoke to Dr. Doering. He hadn't received the report. Apparently, I'm the only who has it. He wants you to meet him at the hospital tomorrow morning at 9:00 a.m. to get to the bottom of the results. He will also have the head of radiology there with him. I won't be there unless you need me to be," she added offering both medical and moral support.

"No. I'll be fine. I trust Dr. Doering. Thanks for watching out for me," I said with my deepest gratitude.

I was stunned that another tumor was growing. It was absolutely beyond me how that was even possible with everything I had been through and done to prevent it, but there it was on the written page. So the cancer was making another run at me.

The following morning, I met Dr. Doering and Dr. Derek, the head of radiology.

"Kathy, Dr. Derek and I have both looked at your scans and are absolutely certain that what Dr. Kerry is calling a new malignancy is really just scar tissue. We don't know why he neglected to look at your history before writing up his report, but he did and that is unforgivable. We are so deeply sorry for his error," Dr. Doering confessed. "You've been through enough and most certainly didn't deserve to be treated that way."

"Would you mind sending me a short letter to make your grievance formal? I know you have enough on your plate, but this will be very helpful for me to discipline Dr. Kerry for his neglect. I am deeply sorry for his mistake and the stress he added to your day," Dr. Derek declared.

It would've been easy to be mad over Dr. Kerry's unprofessional behavior, but I wasn't. I wrote my grievance as requested all the while focusing on the silver lining. I was still cancer free. I hugged my little family before breaking down unexpectedly. From out of nowhere, the darkness of anguish blocked out my silver lining.

Ron held me as I quietly said in his ear, "If it comes back, I just can't do it again!"

He whispered, "I can't imagine."

That mistake, which was ultimately good news, unexplainably sent me over the edge. The following week, I was diagnosed with post-traumatic stress disorder (PTSD) and was sent on another hunt and peck adventure.

March 2008
Dr. Harper asked me to see Dr. Landow, who had been recently hired to start an integrative medicine program at my hospital to help patients using complimentary treatments. In our introductory conversation, I mentioned my recent diagnosis of PTSD, my weight gain and constant fatigue. She skirted the issue of PTSD, seemingly more comfortable discussing something tangible like my thyroid. Dr. Landow explained that Levothyroxine targeted T4, but she wanted me on medicine that went after both the T3 and T4.

She explained that, "the human brain houses the hypothalamus and the pituitary gland, which work together to get the thyroid to function normally. That happens when the hypothalamus sends a message to the pituitary gland in the form of TSH or thyroid stimulating hormone. The pituitary gland takes the TSH and sends that same message to the thyroid to encourage T3 and T4 production. Thyroid cells are the only cells in the body that can absorb iodine, using it with the amino acid tyrosine to produce T4 (thyroxine) and T3 (triiodothyronine). Both are sent into the body to control metabolism."

Dr. Landow continued on by saying, "I think you would benefit by switching to Synthroid. I'll send a note over to Dr. Fickle. I believe changing the medication will take care of your weight gain along with your fatigue. I also think acupuncture and Feldenkrais are good options for you. They can help release the scar tissue, which I firmly believe is having a negative impact on your whole body."

She was right about that but not about the thyroid medicine. Dr. Fickle did not believe the switch would help me but agreed to try it anyway and he was right. I continued to gain weight, was much more tired and suffered from worsening constipation.

I decided to leave my body chemistry for another time and attempted to tackle the PTSD through reiki, meditation and maple syrup production. All three were far more enjoyable than sitting in a therapist's office rehashing the trauma I had suffered. The early spring weather was ripe for the sap to run with daytime temperatures reaching the 40s then dipping down to the 20s at night. The daily freeze and thaw helped the trees pump their sap up through the trunk and into its branches. When we drilled little holes to set our taps, we created a small leak in the system that allowed us to be nourished as well. As we did the previous year, we collected, filtered and boiled the sap down into syrup, filled the bottles, and then wiped them clean before packing them in a cardboard box. I loved the smell of the sap permeating the house, the steam on the windows laden with sugar, and even the sound of my shoes crinkling with each sticky step on the old maple floor. How could I do anything but smile as I admired those jars of amber colored sugar lining my counter. It was indeed therapy for my soul.

Maple syrup season also gave me something more positive to talk about when I found myself in any kind of social situation, which were generally an unbearable challenge for me at the time. It was never more than a few minutes before someone would ask me about my "journey." The use of that word made me cringe. For me, the word journey denoted progression not regression and fighting cancer the conventional way necessarily resulted in at the very least a physical regression, which, in case there is any confusion on that point, was not a good thing. I also defined "journey" as something a person chose to do, an odyssey of sorts. So to call my cancer diagnosis "a journey," was really more for the comfort of others. Perhaps the term was best assigned to the spiritual changes I was experiencing, but then again, those conversations made people uncomfortable. No one wanted to hear about my spiritual progression or journey, but maybe if someone had, I could've engaged in conversation much more easily. Was I over thinking it? Probably, but as I opened up to a deeper spiritual self, my entire being no longer skimmed the surface of life. It was impossible for me to not want to know other people in a more profound way, but that was rarely obliged.

In any case, when the question about my journey was put to me, I launched into a litany of recovery struggles. Even though I had the garden and syrup to talk about, I was programmed, if you will, to start spouting off my list of side effects. It was a trained response by my medical team who, at every appointment asked, "How are you?" expecting me to list which side effects I was still working through. Consequently, conversations in a social setting ended before they even started, because no one wanted to hear about my clogged bowels. They were looking for a customary response like "I'm great" or "Never better." It was emotionally painful to watch the group laughing and enjoying each other as I stood on the side lines hanging on to life by a thread in my somewhat dream-like state and entirely unable to match their revelry. It was useless for me to even attempt to engage because once a conversation had begun, I lost focus and shut down like an infant might do when overstimulated. The noise caused my ear to ache, and while I hated to pull Ron away from the fun, I would inevitably have to for my own preservation.

My girls were the best at keeping me from the depths of despair. During maple syrup season, they begged like baby birds for a spoonful of finished syrup, and with the sun moving closer to the earth and warming the frozen ground, EmmaGrace and Hannah were crazed with playing outside. The biggest laugh they gave me was over a game of tag with the horses. The girls skipped over by the horses, screamed, laughed and ran away. I was convinced that the horses loved the game as much as the girls did. Every time the girls screamed, the horses jumped in the air on cue with their heads down, bucking and chasing EmmaGrace and Hannah through the pasture. I swore they were laughing as hard as the kids, swinging their heads side to side and up and down with the jerking movements of a full belly laugh. I watched the joyous play in the bright sunshine and felt the farm stretch its muscles for another season of growth. I drew the fresh warm air deep into my lungs and let it out with a jubilant sigh. My body embraced the healing power of spring and every one of my cells felt stimulated by the cleansing energy of the earth.

While the girls continued to play, I sat on the deck, completing a list of produce for our garden expansion, which included garlic, onion, sweet potato, potato, leek, radish, lettuce, spinach, chard, garbanzo beans, tomatoes, broccoli, beats, beans, peas, turnips, zucchini, yellow squash, cucumbers, carrots, sweet and spicy peppers, cabbage, celery, oregano, cilantro, basil, tarragon, fennel, chamomile, thyme, sage, lavender, lemon balm, mint, celeriac, sorrel, rosemary, chives, parsley, strawberry, rhubarb, elderberry, blueberries and black raspberries. Many of the flowers I planted were not only beautiful but edible and some like chamomile, borage, calendula, arugula, and my favorite lemon verbena held wonderful healing properties. In total, our expanded garden along with the chickens provided 80% of our food supply and 100% of my rejuvenation. As I burrowed into the farm, I lost touch with friends, and while it seemed like I should feel alarmed by that, I wasn't. My days were filled with a profound sense of peace and growing strength that was entirely addictive.

April 2008
My resolve to fully embrace the healing power of food was intensified one afternoon in the halls of the girls' school where I ran into Kate, a teacher battling cancer. She looked typically frail and while I felt deep compassion for her plight, it was clear she wasn't eating. I wanted to encourage her to eat with the intention to heal, but I knew it wouldn't make a difference. In all honesty, it was clear to me that she would be leaving our earth in the not-so-distant future. Kate shuffled towards me in the hall, then stopped, looking right into my soul with her compassionate eyes. I felt a huge hug exchange between us even though we never touched.

She teared up and said, "We are so fortunate."

I said, "We all have a different path."

She clearly knew what I meant and we exchanged one more mental hug before she continued slowly down the hall. Kate died soon after that, leaving me the gift of an even stronger resolve to go all in with using food as my medicine.

June 2008
Cancer amplified the old adage that "you have to take the good with the bad," and in an effort to keep perspective on where my good vs. bad ratio sat, each morning I listed in my journal what was good about the previous day. It was easy to get caught up in the drama of "bad" events, but if I stayed focused on the "good," I could handle the "bad" a little easier. For example, a new bone scan gave inconclusive results about two spots on my ribs. The spots were either fractures caused by radiation treatment or metastatic cancer. While Dr. Harper explained the divergent opinions on my results, I knew that when they rescanned me in three months, the results would clearly show that the spots were "just" fractures. It was an untenable position, but while the doctors couldn't do anything in that moment, I could. I was moving on from managing

197

cancer conventionally to managing cancer through my gardens, my cooking, my meditative healings and reiki. I was most definitely using a self-prescribed integrative approach, and it seemed to be working. However, it was hard for my doctors to come along for the ride because the medical culture was one of reductionism, having evolved away from looking at the whole person by reducing our needs into specialties.

To that end, my doctors were always searching for trouble. Dr. Harper decided I might have contracted Lupus, a chronic autoimmune disease causing the immune system to attack the body and wanted me tested. As I disengaged from conventional medicine, Lupus didn't even register as a possibility for me. I grew weary of the hunt and peck approach to my health care, which operated on the belief that I "should" be sicker than I was and that just "didn't seem right." I delved even deeper into reiki, meditation and visualization practices and reluctantly exercised to pump oxygen into my blood stream, creating a more aerobic state that would be less appealing to cancer. Since I didn't want to waste my energy eating foods with claims based in pseudo-science, I confirmed that my list of foods had the science to back it up. While it was logical to surmise that other produce could fight cancer as well, I was laser focused on maximizing my benefits and only wanted the foods with proof.

More and more I was asked by other patients why I was doing as well as I was, and after sharing the details of what I was doing, each one of those people took my strategy to their doctors who responded only with ego, "Well, there's no data to back up her claims. Just stay the course." Had their doctors looked into the research, they would've found that there was a strong argument being made to use food as medicine against cancer. Perhaps that little extra effort could've saved the lives of some of those patients.

"People don't resist change; they resist being changed." – Anonymous

Constantly being around death nudged me back towards depression. It took all of my energy, strength and resolve to stay steady for my family, but Aromasin trounced my emotional weakness and altered my mental state. Depression and Aromasin proved to be formidable foes, leading me down the chemically altered path of anger and sadness, which resulted in me snapping at my girls without cause. It was so painful for all of us, especially since they had no way to understand what was happening in my mind and body. What they knew was that they were being let down by the one person who loved them most. I couldn't see how they would still love me if I survived and prayed every day that they would be strong and patient enough to forgive me. I needed them to know deep in their hearts that I loved them more than life itself and couldn't possibly shoulder them resenting me.

"Lord, grant me infinite patience to go with my infinite love."

July 2008
In an attempt to alleviate some of my symptoms, Dr. Harper decided to switch me from Aromasin to Faslodex. My anticipation of reduced side effects was actually met with more. I suffered more migraines, nausea, chills, diarrhea and cramps, which caused me to lay helpless in bed most days. While Ron worked, EmmaGrace sat with me, brought me drinks and watched over five-year old Hannah, all while carrying her veil of sadness everywhere she went. I couldn't imagine what was going through her sweet little mind. EmmaGrace was caring for her mother while being a mother to her little sister. It just wasn't right.

"Would you like to call Grandma," I asked.

She shook her head yes.

"Did the cancer come back?" she asked bracing for the impending dread.

"The medications keeping the cancer away make me feel terrible, and I know some days are worse than others, and it's just awful. I can't even express how sorry I am. I'm incredibly grateful that you are willing to help me out while I work to stay strong," I expressed compassionately.

We were all frustrated, and the promised CLIMB program still hadn't begun. Ron and I struggled to explain what was happening to me, but as hard as I tried to break free, the cancer world kept me bound and gagged.

Since Aromasin hadn't hit me quite as hard as Faslodex, I reluctantly switched back, hoping the fits of rage could be suppressed, but they came back with a vengeance. My brain chemistry was being altered to save my life and I had nowhere to turn. While I desperately wanted to break free from the cancer community, it was my support network and I was woven into its fabric. While the medical professionals encouraged me not to let cancer define me, the fact was that it informed the way I felt, what I thought about and how I spent my time. By design it defined my life, changing it like no other event I had ever experienced. Cancer heightened my awareness of tragedy but also of joy. The

littlest things made me angry, while other tiny things brought overflowing joy. For example, Hannah liked to hold her hand out of the car window with her fingers up in a peace sign.

As we passed cars she yelled, "Peace, Baby. Peace!"

It always came out of the blue and made me wonder if it was somehow another message from the heavens for me to find peace in whatever came my way.

Regeneration

August 2008

Deeper meditations brought deeper revelations. While for a time cancer was the project of my life, I decided it had more importantly become an opportunity for me to learn. I speculated on what I was learning and got lost in the minutia of chasing every little ache or bump that popped up. So much of getting better had become about learning to live in the normal world again, staying in remission with prescription medications or submitting to tests that could cause a third type of cancer to take hold in my weakened body. However, there was something more. My meditation practice was opening me to a wave of change that was coming for me whether I wanted it to or not.

September 2008

CLIMB CLUB finally began, and I was thrilled my girls were going to get some kind of professional help to cope with my diagnosis. The acronym stood for Children's Lives Include Moments of Bravery, and the Club was a workshop series developed by the Children's Treehouse Foundation in Denver, Colorado for kids who had a sibling or parent with cancer. It used art therapy, music and speech to help them work through their feelings. Even though Hannah didn't seem to get very much out of it at five years old, EmmaGrace absorbed it all. One afternoon when we were hanging out together at home, she asked me to draw a picture of what it felt like while I had cancer and she would do the same. Then, she instructed me to draw a picture of what I would feel like if it came back, but I told her I couldn't think about "if it came back" because that would be giving energy to the cancer. She agreed and changed my assignment to drawing how I felt being with her and doing a project. I thought for a moment. I never liked the art therapy sessions because I wasn't very creative in that way, but I tried for her. I illustrated myself as a tree in both cases and EmmaGrace drew herself crying in the first picture and in the second she drew a mosaic of beautiful colors. She labeled our work *A Story Of A Mother and Daughter Going Through Cancer Together.*

"Why did you draw a tree, Mama?" EmmaGrace asked me.

"I don't really know. I suppose because I'm strongly rooted in my family, and even though a tree might lose some big branches, it still lives on because its roots are firmly planted in the ground. I am firmly planted in my family, and when I lost so much fighting cancer, I was still able to live well. I know this to be true especially when I hold you and your sister in my arms."

"Oh, I get it," she said as she closed our drawing books and skittered away.

Later that month, another television station asked to interview me along with Melissa, the counselor responsible for conducting CLIMB CLUB.

"Why did you decide to put your kids in CLIMB?" the reporter asked without any emotion what so ever.

"I signed my daughters up because I thought CLIMB would give them a space to be with other kids and openly discuss how they felt about my battle," I responded, hoping she'd ask me to go deeper.

The reporter didn't ask me anymore questions throughout the rest of the interview, leaving me to sit awkwardly next to Melissa while she explained the ins and outs of the CLIMB workshop. When it was all over and I handed the microphone attached to my shirt back to the camera man, it hit me. I was there as the token cancer patient. They could've done the interview without me, but they wanted a cancer patient on "display" for Melissa.

October 2008
Word continued to spread that I was still alive despite everything I had been through, which led to an overwhelming number of requests to counsel patients like me. For them, my story represented hope, but I struggled to be an example as I listened to their challenges. If cancer returned, what then? Before going too far down that doubtful road, the trip I had been waiting for had finally arrived. It was time for Commonweal and some much needed help. Ron flew with me to San Francisco for a little vacation before he sent me west over the Golden Gate Bridge with the rental car. Driving alone, I felt disoriented as I navigated the treacherously beautiful stretch of Shoreline Highway 1, hugging the cliffs just south of Muir Woods, then regrouping my nerves as I continued to crawl along through Stinson Beach, a bustling resort town at the base of a cliff. I traversed the incline to Mesa Road, turning left towards Commonweal just outside of Bolinas. Before driving all the way up their driveway, I stopped the car and cried. I cried off and on like that for four days, having no control over when it started or when it stopped.

The thoughtfully designed cancer retreat had me taking yoga and meditation classes twice a day with Jnani who was sunshine in human form, individual and group counseling sessions masterfully held by Lenore, and afternoon walks that brought me closer to myself and my fellow participants. There were eight of us in all with 11 staff members carefully attending to our every need over an eight-day period. Michael Lerner, who cofounded the organization with Dr. Remen, led the group discussions at night and one such discussion focused on death and dying. Even though I was mostly convinced I would not die, looking around the room brought that old feeling of fear back stronger than ever. It was hard for me to consider the challenges each of my new friends faced. Mary from Illinois had metastatic triple negative breast cancer, Rosemary from California had bone cancer throughout her entire skeleton, Anna from Russia was in remission from triple negative breast cancer, and Jane from California was battling breast and ovarian cancer coupled with a debilitating autoimmune arthritis. Then, there was sweet Elaina who had colon cancer and an abusive husband.

The food we ate throughout those eight days was anti-inflammatory, organic and purchased from local farmers to nourish our bodies and our souls. On the fifth day, I woke up feeling stronger than I had in years and noticed that the arthritic pain I had lived with since I was 19 years old had faded without the help of medication. I leapt out of bed anxious to do something edgy and set my sights on going where we were instructed not to go – the beach. Laughing joyfully in my single room at the end of the hall, I studied the path outside my window that cut through the woods, over the cliff and down to the beach. We had been asked to stay away from it because it was difficult to navigate, but I felt a piece of my old self surface and set my mind on spending my free time that morning at the water's edge. Before cancer, I was a mountain climber, rock climber, ice climber, wilderness camper and paddler, surely I could get down to the beach.

At breakfast, I chatted with Lenore who instantaneously picked up on my shifted energy.

"Where are you planning on walking this morning," she asked with a sense of already knowing.

My response was weak and evasive, "Oh, I don't know. Maybe over to the cliff's edge."

With a smile, she winked at me.

"Would you like to borrow my tennis shoes? I've noticed you only have sandals here," Lenore asked rhetorically knowing I would have to say yes.

I stood at least eight inches above her, but she wore the same size shoe! Anything seemed possible at Commonweal. I slipped into her black tennis shoes and laced them up quickly, hoping to slip out the front door unnoticed.

As I started to close the door, Lenore stopped its motion with her hand and said, "Be safe where ever it is you're going."

She winked again and closed the door as I stepped off the front porch.

Mindful of mountain lions, I felt like a kid as I skipped down one of the paths in Point Reyes National Seashore. We had been warned that they were in the area, but I felt entirely invincible in that moment and watched for them more out of curiosity than fear. The trail dropped down at the cliff's edge into a small canyon formed by the pounding ocean waves. There was a torn and tattered rope tied between the top and the bottom anchored by rotting wooden posts. That familiar hot surge of adrenaline shot through my body, and just as I began to think better of my plan, a surfer popped up out of nowhere with his black Labrador. He smiled, grabbed the rope without hesitation and dropped down almost like rappelling off a mountain as his dog trailed jubilantly behind. Their enthusiasm was infectious, leaving me no choice but to take a breath and follow suit. I grabbed the rope and descended to the beach in what felt like one fluid motion. At the bottom, I trotted to the water's edge feeling elated and couldn't remember the last time I had felt that way. At the shoreline, I found the wet dog watching his surfer navigate the waves, but when he saw me, it was like we were old friends. He bounded towards me with a stick between his jaws and tail wagging like the needle on a metronome. I lost track of time on that beach and permanently reclaimed another little piece of myself while I rediscovered the happiness I had previously surrendered to cancer. I felt so proud of my accomplishment but told no one. Change was no longer on the wind for me, it had arrived through little incremental victories, and for the first time since being diagnosed, I cried tears of indescribable joy.

Prior to cancer, advocacy was at my core. I worked in it, lived in it and chronically volunteered in it from my preteen years on. After my diagnosis, I abandoned it all, and while I tried to advocate for myself, I also allowed myself to be stripped of who I was, letting the treatment and subsequent drugs leave me a shell of my former self. At Commonweal, the word and concept of advocacy showed up during every meditation and sand tray session I had. At a soul level I knew what it meant, but I pushed it off. Being an advocate was a terribly difficult job made much harder by the emotional passion I had for justice on all levels. So the idea that I would have the strength to go back to advocating, seemed laughable at best. Fortunately, I couldn't suppress who I was and the spirit within me resurfaced, compassionately coaxing me back towards my intended path.

I was already practicing eating with the intention to heal before I had arrived, but none of the other participants were. They appeared to be in a weaker state than I was and struggled with the disease fighting menu presented each day. I was passionate about their survival just as I was for the other patients I had met over the previous three years, and it got me thinking. I turned my meditations towards teaching how to eat with the intention to heal. I had no clear vision at that point, but I could feel its glow. On the eighth day, I left the womb of

Commonweal empowered to act. My time there was the spark that reignited the entrepreneurial spirit within me, and several months later, I started a non-profit organization focused on using food as medicine but more on that later.

November 2008
Another set of PET and CT scans delivered another set of results confirming that I was still cancer free, which left another set of doctors questioning how it was even possible. At that point, they weren't interested in how I got there, they were more inclined to believe my recovery was a fluke. So instead of engaging their misdirected questions, I celebrated the results with my dogs and headed for the top of our hill where I planted my feet and ejected my accumulated stress through a piercing war cry followed by a high-pitched howl that sent the dogs into a frenzy, jumping and yipping in unison around my feet.

"We are blessed!!" I yelled as I threw my arms up to the heavens. "Thank you, Lord!"

November brought additional reconstructive surgery from which I contracted yet another infection in my right breast. However, I was much quicker to push back by honing in on the positives even though fatigue, anger and constipation still lingered like the plague at the door of my recovering body. I clung to the good and rejected the drama of the bad, embracing every silver lining that came my way. Overlooking the infection, I found gratitude for Dr. Sanders who had removed the entanglement of scar tissue twisting my rib cage and released the lace work of scars that dragged my arm pit halfway to my elbow. When he released those two areas, he brought indescribable relief to my body just in time for another Thanksgiving dinner with our families. We hosted again that year, and my favorite part of the evening was when we shared what we were thankful for.

During my turn, I looked up to the ceiling and said, "I am grateful for the strength God has given me to endure the onslaught of treatments and barrage of emotional pitfalls while still leaving me something left to climb back up onto the mesa of me."

December 2008
The Christmas season always brought an overload of wonderment to our days, but that year was especially compelling for me. I had been spared but was far from unscathed. I had accepted what I believed to be the illuminated path God had sent me down and honored His plan by making a decision that was both comforting and intimidating. I had decided to jump the protocol ship for good and would no longer be taking Aromasin or any other cancer drug. It was time for me to do the herculean task of freeing myself from lymphedema, bone pain,

headaches, nausea, fatigue, acid reflux, hot flashes, compromised kidneys, decreased lung capacity, constipation, bloating, loss of intestinal function and rage. In all honesty it was the loss of intestinal function and continuous rage that broke this camel's back, tipping the scales in favor of moving away from the slippery slope of medical protocols, and making it crystal clear that whether I lived or died I needed my children to love me and for them to know I loved them.

Sitting on the exam table in a cotton hospital gown at eye level with Dr. Harper, I set my sight squarely on his eyes and said with complete conviction, "It really seems like all the drugs I've been taking only weaken my body more. I need to feel strong again, so I'm going to dedicate myself to solely using foods with antiangiogenic properties together with reiki and meditative practices to stay in remission and continue to heal. I hope you understand."

"I understand where you're coming from, but you can understand why I disagree with this approach. There just isn't enough data to support your choice, but if you are determined, I'll continue on with you and we'll see how it goes," Dr. Harper responded with genuine concern. "It's going to take about two weeks to flush your system of all of the drugs. So, just keep that in mind."

I left the cancer clinic energized by being unencumbered from conventional medicine, and elated that reiki, yoga, meditation and mindfulness would become the bedrock of my daily routine.

January 2009

After dropping Aromasin, certain side effects escalated as I purged the remaining toxins like the final heave of a dying body. It became painfully clear that even though I was no longer taking the cancer meds, my body was still in decline from their long-term effects. Headaches came in full force, my heart function was failing, and water engorged my every cell like a rubber balloon filled at the tap. My body packed on an impossible six pounds in one week, and while the specific cause was unclear, the treatment was well known to Dr. Fickle. To protect my damaged heart, he swiftly put me on Spironolactone, a diuretic that would reduce the fluid around my heart while wringing out the water from the rest of my tissue like a sponge. In only a couple of weeks, I dropped close to 20 pounds of water weight, stood up straighter and felt more like my old self than I had in years. Even though it was a new medication, I was grateful for the relief and knew I would be able to stop taking it someday.

With another issue resolved, I turned to my erratic thyroid seemingly not willing to be tamed by the wide range of ArmourThyroid doses I had been subjected to. Recognizing that we weren't really getting anywhere, Dr. Fickle sent me to a specialist by the name of Dr. Petri, who was considered to be the best endocrinologist in Wisconsin at that time. At our first meeting, it was clear he was very smart. Dr. Petri came into the room looking like every other doctor I had met, but his awkward behavior was revealed almost immediately. He put his note pad down on the little desk attached to the requisite exam room cabinets, sat down and stared at them as he mumbled something about how nice it was to meet me. He never actually looked at me when he said it, and each time he repeated that same phrase in the same way throughout my appointment, he left me questioning the stability of his mind. Dr. Petri performed an abbreviated physical exam and asked if he could look at my driver's license to see what I looked like before I was diagnosed. What he was able to see from the picture was never revealed to me and his 'technique' seemed like more of a quirk in his protocol than anything else. He signed me up for a sleep study and changed my medication from Armour Thyroid back to levothyroxine.

I explained, "I was put on Armour Thyroid because it was more natural than levothyroxine."

Dr. Petri responded, "It's only natural if you're a pig. Are you a pig?"

I looked at him with a raised eyebrow and he caught my meaning immediately, shifting his tone and moving on to a more medical explanation. He said the pig hormone may be good for pigs, but it's not necessarily always good for people. I forgave his first response in hopes that he would offer something useful in my quest for the Holy Grail of a renewed metabolic system.

"I'm going to have you submit to blood work to evaluate your hormones. Just wait here and Lisa will come and get you," Dr. Petri commanded.

That was it. There was no good-bye, no thanks for choosing me, no I'll call you with the results. He just walked out without saying a word.

When Lisa arrived to lead me to Dr. Petri's shiny new lab, I felt flushed with adrenaline. It was that feeling you get when you're home alone at night and you hear a noise that makes every sensor in your body prickle with fear. Needless-to-say, needles were a trigger for my PTSD. So when the phlebotomist appeared carrying a stainless-steel tray laden with alcohol pads, Band-Aids, cotton swabs, a blue tourniquet and a needle, I blanched and took in a gulp of air as if she had startled me.

Ignoring my obvious fear, the phlebotomist asked, "Is there an arm you prefer?"

Pausing for a minute with my hands under my thighs, I looked down at the floor and then slowly raised my left arm, quietly answering, "I have lymphedema in my right arm."

She took my left arm, pushed my sleeve up above my elbow and began to prepare the area on the inside of my elbow for the jab.

"No! You can't do it there. The veins are scarred and hard to find. You need to get a butterfly needle and do it on top of my hand," I demanded surprising even myself.

The phlebotomist gave me an odd look and then her eyebrows raised, signaling that she understood. The very tiny needle typically used on children had rubber butterfly wings attached on either side, which made it look more friendly than the others. More importantly, it provided a grip, giving the phlebotomist better control. She easily slid the needle into the large vein on the top of my hand and drained eight vials of blood before handing me an empty tube.

"You are to spit in this tube at precisely 11:00 p.m. tonight. Tomorrow morning, put it in this pre-stamped tube and drop it in the mail," she instructed without any perceivable emotion.

Several days later, Dr. Petri called to say that he had assessed every hormone in my body including cortisol but found nothing of note, except for the liver disease revealed in my blood work.

Without thinking about who I was talking to I said, "Isn't liver disease worth noting."

"Of course, but it's not the cause of your other issues. I'll send a report to Dr. Fickle. Good bye," Dr. Petri concluded before abruptly hanging up the phone.

Ultimately without any help from Dr. Petri, Dr. Fickle got my thyroid levels in balance by alternating the use of two different doses of Levothyroxine throughout the week.

After the call with Dr. Petri, I decided to look through my old work files, hoping to reconnect with the person I was before cancer picked up my life and dumped it out all over the floor. I flipped through old newspaper clippings in which I had been interviewed, read through speeches I had given and sorted through work I had produced. The common theme of my life had been trying to make the world a better place, and it was a good reminder of what I was made to do. Soon after that reminder, I ran into Barb, the executive director of the cancer center. I took advantage of the opportunity and requested a meeting to discuss my thoughts around how to help other cancer patients do as well as I had.

"I would really like to hear about what you're thinking. Would you mind if I invite some other key decision makers to our meeting?" Barb asked respectfully.

"Oh! Of course not," I responded feeling absolutely delighted.

In that tiny moment, Barb had validated me and for that I will be ever grateful. She reminded me that my ideas were worthy of hearing. Later that day, my elevated attitude was challenged by a call from my good friend and Commonweal Comrade Mary Utne O'Brien. She called to tell me her cancer had spread to her liver and spine. I was devastated for her and wanted nothing more at that moment than for her to be where I was, three years and three months out from diagnosis, gripping clean pet scans. If anyone deserved to be free of the beast, it was Mary, and while my scans were clean, her news affirmed that the fear of recurrence was etched deep in my cells.

Just after Mary's call, EmmaGrace asked for help with math, but as soon as I began to read the instructions with her, I was forced to excuse myself to the den where a deluge of tears and emotions submerged my brightening spirit. I cried uncontrollably until EmmaGrace appeared by my side, comforting me by rubbing my back just as I had done for her countless times before. The compassion in EmmaGrace's tiny hands helped me regain control and apologize for interrupting her homework.

The next morning, I was up at the crack of dawn to meet with Dr. Doering for coffee. I told him of my impending meeting with Barb and asked if I could run my thoughts by him to be sure they were coherent. We discussed how ProHealth Care could make a huge shift in cancer treatment by adopting a companion practice of using food as medicine.

As I handed Dr. Doering the one-page summary I had painstakingly prepared, he stared right in my eyes and said, "I'm sorry we weren't able to help you with preventing lymphedema. Today, we would do better."

I smiled and continued to discuss my desire to teach food as medicine along with creating a garden for patients like me to tend or stroll through as desired. My hope was that the garden would be large enough to provide produce to feed patients in the hospital.

"I like that a lot. I grew up on a farm and really do believe what you are talking about. Would you be willing to speak about your plan at our directors meeting as my guest? I know Barb has you already booked for a meeting with some other decision makers, but this would be a great group for you to pitch your idea," Dr. Doering requested with an encouraging smile.

I agreed even though the idea was admittedly intimidating. I was still struggling to put words together in a coherent sentence but noticed the more I engaged conversation the easier it got. Once our short conversation had concluded, I thanked my surgeon for taking the time to talk with me and handed him a bottle of our maple syrup along with a copy of the *ANTICANCER* book.

February 2009
February found me back in the hospital with severe constipation, a slight fever and more pain in my abdomen. Dr. Fickle ordered tests, which found nothing. A few days later, I was back in the ER with an even higher fever and much more pain. A small bowel test was ordered that required me to obediently drink a thick white liquid called barium. Then the radiologist watched it move through my intestines on the x-ray screen. After several minutes, a large mass appeared and the machine stayed on it until it dislodged like a clog in a sink drain. Dr. Harrison, the radiologist, concluded that something was causing my intestines to malfunction and an exploratory surgery was in order with Dr. Doering doing the honors.

During the surgery, Dr. Doering removed extensive adhesions that had ensnared my intestines presumably interfering with their motility. He also stumbled upon endometriosis, which also could have been the source of the adhesions. At the end of my surgery, Dr. Doering concluded that the source of my constipation was definitely a lack of motility in my intestinal muscle, but it was not caused by adhesions. It was most likely caused by Aromasin and unfortunately, my intestines may never recover. Being one of the largest organs in the human body, intestines work to strengthen the immune system by absorbing nutrients and water in one action and moving waste products out of the body in another. Since my intestinal tract wasn't doing the later, I was immediately prescribed an intense regimen of various laxatives. From that point on, each morning and evening, I took a double dose of polyethylene glycol, along with a 500-mg chaser of magnesium citrate, and added a double shot of Milk of Magnesia before bed. It quickly became obvious that their cumulative effects were unpredictable at best, leaving me no choice but to remain flexible. I adjusted my days by never leaving the house before 10:00 a.m., which brought with it the silver lining benefit of time to refocus on the gift of my ordeal and move full steam ahead to fully develop my ideas around teaching in the hospital.

While it felt daunting to create a synopsis of the program I wanted to teach, I reminded myself that I had pulverized two different types of cancer. Surely, creating a food as medicine program would be easier than that. Ahead of our meeting, Barb sent out an email with a list of invitees that gave me a "holy crap they really are taking me seriously" moment. It wasn't just an "appeasement of the patient" type of meeting it was the real deal. They had opened their doors wide to me and I was going to walk through no matter what. My vision was a program that would help support patients through cancer and potentially help them prevent recurrence. It would have to be a community effort if we were going to save lives and I was truly committed to making that happen. I presented my thoughts at the meeting and enjoyed support around the table with one exception. Dr. Johnson, whose work focused on diabetes. He was dubious about using food as medicine. Yes, that's right. Your thoughts are exactly what I thought. 'Ummmmm, a doctor who works with diabetics didn't like the idea of using food as medicine?'

His comments were something along the lines of, "I'm uncomfortable telling people to use food as medicine because we don't know what food will do or how it will interact with their medication."

I had to pick my jaw up from the floor, wondering if in fact he had said what I thought he had.

My first response was, "Ummmmmmmm," before pulling myself together and explaining, "It's time to do something different. Let me remind you that prescription medications were given to me without any real understanding of their interactions with each other or the impacts they would have on me. As a result, I have suffered way beyond what I believe was necessary. Using food as medicine in conjunction with meditation and energy work has brought me nothing but healing. Wouldn't you agree that it's a huge stretch to put fresh whole foods in the same category as synthesized drugs."

His response? Nothing.

March 2009
By all counts except for Dr. Johnson's, the meeting went well. Barb wrote him a "Dear, John" letter and then asked me to speak at the ProHealth Care leadership conference in April with the goal of sharing my perspective on what their system did right and what it did wrong for me. Admittedly, I was stunned by her request and asked if she really meant for me to outline what they had done "wrong." Confirming that it was exactly what she meant, Barb was thrilled that I agreed and ended our conversation with an "Oh, by the way," report that there would be nearly 500 leaders at the event. That number threw

me for a loop. I silently scolded myself for my insecurities because I had spoken to groups more than twice that size in the past, but while the battle with cancer had brought me strength, it also left behind insecurity. I wrote my speech, rehearsed it over and over in the mirror and then enlisted Ron and my dad to accompany me to the conference. After I was introduced, I told my story through jittery nerves, praised my doctors, critiqued the system, and made recommendations for improvement. At the conclusion, I was overwhelmed by a standing ovation and an invitation to meet with the CEO, Ford Titus, who was a true visionary and deeply committed to his community. Being there was an energy rush for me and another validation of the direction I was headed in.

I continued to use reiki to further heal and balance my energy fields just like a pacemaker balanced the electrical impulses of the heart. I meditated multiple times throughout the and sometimes with the intention of better understanding my path. I questioned whether starting an educational program around eating with the intention to heal, was where my efforts were needed, and on several occasions, my heart heard "write a book instead." Although, I loved the idea of writing, I ignored the guidance and stubbornly stayed on the path of working in the hospital.

April 2009
April brought spring to our farm, signaling another growing season. I organized boxes of seeds on my dining room table and drew a diagram depicting where they would be planted. The girls admired the seed packets taking each one out of its box to study the picture on the front, leaving them awestruck that such a large fruit or vegetable could come from such a tiny little seed. When the young plants arrived, we carried them out to the garden in an almost reverent procession. Ron had created a bed specifically for the three-year-old asparagus roots we had purchased. An asparagus patch is a long-term investment, and even though the roots were three years old, they were not likely to produce harvestable stalks for at least a year. I dug small holes in one row for the girls to carefully place the strawberry plants. In another bed, they helped me plant the raspberry, black berry, blueberry and elderberry saplings, holding them while I covered the roots with dirt and tamped them down. We stood back and admired each plant that would garner powerful cancer fighting compounds for us as they grew.

June 2009
With the garden in full bloom and nearing harvest, I directed my attention back to scheduling a meeting with Ford Titus. When I called his assistant Mary, I was pleasantly surprised by her warm greeting. Ford was confident that I would call and had given her the heads up for which I was very grateful. During the meeting, Ford was equally as warm and his gracious demeanor diffused my

nervousness, freeing me to easily discuss my ideas for his non-profit hospital. He especially liked the idea of growing food, serving it in his cafeteria and teaching patients how to cook it at home. Where we parted ways, was in the creation of a nonprofit organization. Having spent my entire career in the non-profit world, the last thing I wanted to do was start a new one, but Ford was steadfast. He would be retiring in 2011 and wanted my project to have a life beyond his retirement. He rightly believed the new CEO would cut any whole food education and might even cut the integrative medicine program he had launched. I came to learn that Ford most definitely had the gift of foresight because the CEO who followed him did exactly what he had predicted, showing a complete lack of understanding for where health care was going in exchange for adding profits to the bottom line.

Although my meditations continued to produce counsel against it, I moved forward with Ford. In 2009, we set up our board and in 2010, we incorporated as NuGenesis Farm and harvested our first crops. In 2011, we received non-profit status to support a farming education center focused on scientifically confirmed foods that fought widespread chronic illness, and by 2014, we enjoyed countless volunteer hours graciously given by more than 1,000 people. Each of those volunteers helped to realize my vision by working to establish the organization, teach about sustainable agriculture, catalyze research around food as medicine and demonstrate cooking techniques that retained the nutritional benefits of food. My hope was that we would someday work ourselves out of business, having also served as an incubator for others to start their own businesses around the principles of using food as medicine. In 2016, NuGenesis closed its doors. During its tenure, NuGenesis trained dietitians, teachers, chefs, farmers, students,corporations, medical practitioners and the public while also serving as a job training site for Easter Seals and The Center for Independent Living. It was humbling for me to understand that the fear of cancer motivated people from all walks of life to come together and make a change.

While I was chugging along with running an organization, raising my kids, and trying to recover from cancer treatment, my dad was diagnosed with esophageal cancer. That started the whole process all over again for my family. He had gone to his doctor earlier in the year because of acid reflux, during which time he was given a prescription for Omeprazole to help manage it. Unfortunately, what his doctor neglected to mention was that acid reflux could lead to or indicate esophageal cancer. My Dad's doctor failed him a second time by not referring him to a gastroenterologist who would have tested him for Gerd and Barrett's esophagus along with cancer. If my dad had been diagnosed with Gerd or Barrett's, the omeprazole would likely have healed his esophagus, preventing cancer from developing. Since none of that was explained to my dad, who didn't like to take medicine, he decided not to take it. By June, a five

213

centimeter tumor was found, and believing it was still operable, Dr. Harper sent him for surgery at the University of Wisconsin – Madison Hospital and Clinics. Unfortunately, the surgeon there delayed my dad's surgery for a few weeks, claiming that it wouldn't matter for the cancer, but it did.

I desperately explained to my dad that, "a two-centimeter tumor can shed over two million cancer cells a day, quickly spreading the disease. Your tumor is double that size and could shed at least twice that much. Dad, you really can't afford to wait. If you want me to, I'll call the clinic and get you an earlier surgery date."

To my chagrin, he accepted the delay.

I recalled the words of Mary Utne O'Brien who said, "His cancer is not your cancer."

When the surgeon at the university finally did open my dad up, the tumor had grown, penetrating his esophageal wall and wrapping itself around his aortic artery, making surgery impossible. She closed him up, inserted a feeding tube (which was not requested nor was it needed at that time) and sent him home where he battled infection after infection at the site of the tube.

I did my best to pop in on my parents and size up where I could help or just sit and chat, and on one such day after taking a sizeable dose of Lorazepam, my dad confessed that he had asked for the cancer.

"Excuse me? What?" I asked.

"I told God that if he was going to give you more cancer, then I wanted him to give it to me instead. I wished I had been more helpful to you while you were going through it. If I can take it from you, then I would feel like I had done something for you, Honey," he said completely serious.

Now my dad was a well-known joker, but he wasn't joking. Taking cancer intended for me was clearly his coup de grâce against The Plan. His statement left me shocked and speechless.

Then as gently as I could I said, "Dad, I don't believe that's how God works. You did so much for me and my family and not just during the years I was sick. You're a wonderful father and grandfather, not to mention all the wonderful things you've done for others over your life time. No, God did not give you cancer instead of giving it to me. I firmly believe that God is benevolent and not a deal maker."

"Well, I can only tell you what I know," my dad said closing his eyes and squeezing my hand before letting it drop.

There was no helping him understand that diet accounts for the majority of esophageal cancer diagnoses and his was most likely the culprit.

July 2009
Through meditation and mindfulness practices, I opened myself to the enjoyment of everything around me. Most days, I sat on the screened in porch listening to the morning break and watching the sun light up the sky, signaling the rooster to crow. The birds sang out from nearby branches, mourning doves whistled as they fluttered past me on their way to the barn, and my Irish wolfhound lounged in the sand box near my growing garden.

August 2009
In August, I began to give presentations during which I would recite my newly adopted motto: Prevent Cancer, Support Your Body Through Treatment and Prevent Recurrence Using Food As Medicine. Weekly, I met with a variety of people at various stages of their battle, and with each story, my heart broke a little more. Being around so much cancer was taking its toll. I focused on how I could help and ignored my own fragile state. Starting a new organization was beating me down, but it was impossible for me not to finish what I had started. So meeting after meeting, talk after talk, I moved closer to fully implementing NuGenesis. Ford, recognizing its potential, gave it a home on an unused piece of hospital land with a dilapidated house and barn. I embraced his gift and went to work. Peggy, who had lost her sister to cancer also embraced my vision and seized on recruiting contractors to donate their time to renovate the house. Her feat was truly extraordinary. With most of the furnishings provided by Steinhafel's in Waukesha we were up and running. Matt Wade, the facilities manager at the hospital, worked with Ron and I to prepare the land for a community garden. I brought our tractor over and tilled the fields while Matt, among other things, coordinated Eagle Scouts to clear the old debris from the site. We began meetings with architects to design a building and planted our first crops the following spring. It should have been an exhilarating time for me with so many impressive hands working to carry out my plans, but it wasn't. To do the project justice, I had to give up time with my girls and I found that impossible to reconcile.

I economized the hours by developing NuGenesis programs based on my own teaching techniques at home with the girls and used my garden and recipes as a model for its educational programs. When I cooked, I creatively stuffed as many vegetables into one meal as possible to maximize the healing benefits of each bite. For example, I mixed corn, onions and kale together with a little

215

butter, salt and pepper and dubbed it "Packer Corn" as a nod to Ron's family heritage. His Great Uncle Tubby Bero was on the first Packer team and his Grandfather Arthur Bero, a humble cobbler, was one of its first fundraisers back in 1919. I felt like I had scored a touchdown as my girls greedily ate three servings of vegetables at once in the name of family legacy. In my tacos, I mixed Swiss chard, spinach, carrots, onions, garlic, beans, leeks and whatever else I had on hand. In the morning, it was breakfast burritos made from our chickens'eggs along with a variety of chopped vegetables from our garden. I personally needed to take in at least 10 servings a day to keep cancer at bay and my family happily joined in. Since I primarily used ingredients I had on hand, I became known as the "Refrigerator Chef."

September 2009
EmmaGrace's 11th birthday had arrived and U2 was playing in Chicago. Since she had never seen Larry perform, I decided to take her to the concert. He made it into the event of a life time, making her feel like a little rock star as she followed him around like a duckling. Larry organized a room for us down the hall from his at the Trump Tower and made our boondoggle even more exciting when we got to go to the top of the tower. Little Emma Grace was on top of the world. I, on the other hand, was terrified the entire time. Larry, with EmmaGace in tow, went too close to the edge for my liking, and there were no railings to stop them from plunging to their deaths, God forbid. I smiled through my fear and didn't breathe until we were back inside and on the elevator going down to Larry's car. We rode with him to the concert where we were well cared for after our legendary friend peeled off to get ready for the show. The whole experience was wonderfully overwhelming for EmmaGrace who was absolutely awestruck by her very own security detail, and heart-warming for me since I hadn't seen her that happy in ages.

As NuGenesis appeared more often in the local news, my schedule filled up with a multitude of speaking engagements. Even though I was tired, I had pledged to myself that when a door opened, I was going to walk through even if I had no idea where it would lead. In all cases, it was a great experience. I discovered that I really enjoyed sharing my story, which usually opened others to share theirs. Quite often, I was approached after my speech by someone who would say, "I really never talk about my cancer, but…"

While the cancer hadn't killed me, I thought NuGenesis just might. My little project grew like Jack's little seed, turning into a giant bean stalk. Supported by the community, my responsibilities grew to include writing website content, developing marketing materials and educational programs, fundraising, farming, managing a board along with an ever growing population of volunteers, capped off by speaking throughout the community and participating

216

in publicity events. My title was CEO, Board President, Executive Director, Development Director, Program Manager, Volunteer Coordinator and Farmer, and at the same time, I was taking care of my girls and my parents, going to my Dad's appointments, making calls for him, and just trying to be present in any way I could. As you might imagine, my daily meditation and mindfulness practices waned.

I was fully consumed and certain that the stress was going to get me, but somehow each scan and blood draw I underwent offered evidence of my improving health. Some called me lucky to be alive, but I didn't feel so much lucky as drained. I had lost the rhythm of my life and began to feel depression creep back in. Even though I really had earned a break after working so hard to survive and thrive, I couldn't keep what I had learned to myself. Something deep inside forced me to take my story to anyone who would listen and show that there was indeed hope. I believed that beating back cancer or whatever chronic illness we were up against, necessarily had to include eating with the intention to heal. I knew that we could all live better, if we lived better informed.

October 2009
While I stopped paying attention to my own emotional state of decline, one of my friends hadn't. Sheila, invited me to her condo in Jackson Hole, Wyoming to get out into the healthy air of the Grand Teton Mountains. Our first hike was an eye-opener for me even though we decided to take it easy on that first day. We hiked around the hill at the ski resort, and I was so slow compared to Sheila that I was embarrassed by holding her back. She patiently slowed her pace during my frequent stops and finally hitched a ride down the mountain for us from a maintenance worker at the ski resort.

As we bumped our way along the cat tracks, he randomly piped up and said, "Spring and summer in Jackson is for the newlyweds and fall is for the nearly dead."

I guessed that his comment was for my benefit, but he had no idea how accurate he was. Instead of shrinking, I resolved to try harder the next day. On day two, Sheila picked some easier trails by Jenny Lake and I bustled along behind her while listening and watching for grizzly bears. I couldn't shake the thought that it would be just my luck to beat cancer only to be eaten by a bear.

January 2010
New research brought new foods to my diet, and Dr. Jack Losso sent me a bottle of black cumin seed oil, also known as kalonji oil. Made from the seeds of the Nigella sativa black cumin flower, kalonji oil was used as a spice in

217

Middle Eastern cooking. Jack and others had been testing its effectiveness against cancer and found it to be promising even in tackling pancreatic cancer cells. Since I was in remission, he instructed me to take a half a teaspoon daily in my orange juice. The oil had a rancid flavor and foul smell but was made much more palatable when taken with orange or cranberry juice. I took it obediently until it was gone and then ordered more online, reminding myself that when a door opened, I was to walk through.

March 2010
In the midst of the mayhem of my life, a new round of headaches took hold, which obviously meant more scans on which a new challenge was revealed. A nasal polyp that was seen on previous scans had doubled in size. Dr. Harrison whisked me in for endoscopic sinus surgery at Madison, deciding to couple it with a septoplasty, fixing the deviated septum I was left with after breaking my nose 20 years earlier. It was another quick "procedure" that found no cancer, but a surgery none-the-less, emphasizing how much harder it had become for me to recover from the anesthesia each time I went under.

June 2010
My Dad's health was on the decline and one afternoon while I was being interviewed by a local television station at NuGenesis, my mom called and left a message. An hour went by before I was able to listen to it, which left me devastated by the desperation in her voice. My dad had fallen in the shower and she was unable to pick him up. When I didn't answer her call, she was forced to dial 911. The ambulance took my dad to the hospital for a full evaluation during which they gave him fluids for extreme dehydration. I was talking to the cameras in their time of need, and even now, I hate to think about how I let them down.

August 2010
My dad died 14 months after he was diagnosed, and in his last days, he whispered to me that he was not afraid to go, he just didn't want to leave his family. He was uncharacteristically quiet during that time, rarely speaking and when he did we could barely make out what he was saying. On the day he died, the girls and I were with him, trying one last time to squeeze a little more life out of his debilitated body. They danced, sang, and told him stories, hoping to hear his hearty laugh once more. I held his hand and laughed for him, searching his face for any sign that he could hear them, and he could. It was ever so subtle, but I saw the corner of his mouth curve up slightly. There was no mistaking it as a smile.

I leaned my body over his, hugging him and said, "I love you, Dad."

218

"Thank you," he pushed out of his throat quieter than a whisper.

At about 4:30 p.m. while I rested my head on my Dad's bed and held his hand I heard his voice loud and clear, "Take the girls home."

My head shot up and I stared at his blank face. Even though his eyes were closed and his mouth was too dry for any words to form, I knew it was him.

I studied his face intently and asked, "Did you just say that?"
There was no response, not even a slight twitch.

A moment later, my mom was at my side, touching my arm and quietly whispering, "You should take the girls home."

Confused, I asked, "Did you just say that?"

"No," she quietly responded and then drifted back to her chair.

When I asked her later that day, she had no memory of that moment, leaving me convinced that it was my dad speaking through her. I gathered the girls and sent them to my dad one last time before driving home, but no sooner had we walked in the door when my sister called. She was at the house with my mom and reported that my dad drew his last breath moments after we had left. The girls and I raced back to my mom and I held her close.

Through her tears she said, "I just know how lucky I was to have him for so long. I'm okay."

She wasn't okay. I knew that, but I also knew how lucky I was to have such a strong, graceful and loving mother. I had no doubt that it was her mental strength coursing through my veins, keeping me from ever surrendering to the beast.

October 2010
Some days it took everything I had to keep it together. There were the constant complications of being a cancer patient, the loss of my dad along with so many friends, the stress of running an organization while being a mom, and the stress of knowing I had lost myself in the midst of it all. I was hanging on to the edge of a cliff by my fingernails, scratching for the skills I had learned at Commonweal just one year before. I developed bronchitis and pneumonia, and subjected to yet another series of scans, which were all clear of metastases but sent my doctors on another search and rescue operation. A follow-up blood test showed I was in stage III kidney disease and once again suffering from hepatic

steatosis or fatty liver disease caused by the chemotherapy agents I had taken. Staying away from prescription drugs meant turning to Tobins, my family owned community pharmacy with a heavy emphasis on complimentary medicine. Dave, a pharmacist and one of the owners, set me up with milk thistle and dandelion root to help regenerate new liver cells and it worked. My liver recovered.

January 2011
Dr. Harper was worried about my lipid panel and sent me to Lipidologist Dr. Tinsdale. I didn't think to ask my other doctors what they thought, but I should have. She diagnosed me with borderline diabetes, heart disease and metabolic syndrome, putting the fear of God in me and sending me on my way with Niaspan, Metformin and Lovaza. She also suggested I take Crestor, but I drew a line in the sand. As I was leaving her office laden with prescriptions, one of the nurses stopped me.

"I know I'm out of line here, but please go and get a second opinion," she urged. "Dr. Tinsdale tends to, umm overprescribe."

I spoke with a family practice doctor I knew socially who confided that he had worked with her before she was forced out of the practice. He reviewed my labs and completely disagreed with her assessment. Alarmed, I took my results to Dr. Fickle for the final word and he agreed that Dr. Tinsdale had prescribed medicine for a fictitious problem. I was flabbergasted. Apparently, having medical bills well over $600,000, not to mention the potential side effects accompanying each drug she prescribed, wasn't enough for her to more closely scruitinize her proposed "treatment." Soon after, a report was made known to me that outlined how she was paid to speak by the very drug companies whose products she was pushing in her clinic. So for her own personal gain, she had prescribed medication I didn't need.

April 2011
As hard as I tried to stay positive, the debris left by cancer treatment weighed me down. Painfully bloodshot eyes, extreme fatigue and muscle spasms fed my constant need for reassurance that cancer was not coming back. The deaths of people close to me cast a dark cloud over my own prognosis, making it hard to not revisit whether I'd be next. Despite everything I was doing to recover, cancer still had a solid psychological grip on me. There were just too many people who had recurred after an "all clear" from their doctors to sit back on my laurels. Every little ache or pain was suspect and cause for alarm. Then, Dr. Gary Stoner threw his hat in my ring and encouraged me to add black raspberry powder for extra insurance. How could I not? After all, it was functional food carrying no side effects and showing great potential to kill cancer.

May 2011
Friday the 13th was a lucky day for me on the cancer front with the next set of CT and bone scans unable to detect cancer anywhere in my body. However, before I was able to get too excited, the scans did expose dense calcification in my left anterior descending artery. Dr. Harper was as stunned as I was since the cardiogram from five months earlier showed a normally functioning heart. It was clear that Adriamycin chemotherapy, notorious for causing heart damage, had finally made its mark, and if there was a silver lining, I sure couldn't find it. Dr. Harper made a new addition to my team by calling on Cardiologist Dr. Carter, and I made my way to a new department in the hospital. At my appointment with Dr. Carter, he asked about my symptoms. He hadn't gotten too far down his list before I realized he was reading symptoms that were generally associated with a heart attack: heavy chest – check; back pain – check; fatigue – check; nausea/vomiting – check; and dizzy – check. It was clear that my challenges were not over. Following that first appointment, I submitted to a stress test during which he measured the ejection fraction rate (EFR) of my heart, which told him how well my heart was pumping with each beat. During that test, my heart measured in at 42, meaning 42% of the total amount of blood in my left ventricle was being pushed out with each heartbeat. An EFR of less than 40 could indicate heart failure and I was dangerously close, leaving Dr. Carter to order another invasive test, the angiogram. While the results were obviously disappointing, they were also a call to action and a reminder that I could affect the outcome of the next test.

I refocused my energy on healing my heart over the following week, meditating and doing reiki to beat the band. I sent out a plea for help from other practitioners and settled in to knowing that my heart was going to be fine. After more than a week, I underwent the angiogram, during which Dr. Carter made a small slit in my groin to snake a catheter into my femoral artery. Once it was in place, he injected iodine dye and then watched for it to show up on the x-ray monitor as it made its way through my blood stream. The purpose of the angiogram was to look for any blockage in my arteries, namely the previously identified calcification, but my results were curious. Dr. Carter found no calcification in my arteries - anywhere. None at all. Zip, zero, nada. He remarked how strange that was, offering no medical explanation for how the calcification seen on the CT scan was no longer there. In addition, my heart's ejection fraction rate was almost 10 points higher. I believed I knew why but said nothing. The improvement still wasn't great, but it was better. Even so, Dr. Carter felt that he had no choice but to prescribe a drug called Coreg, which he insisted I'd be on forever.

June 2011
I continued to build NuGenesis, working to make it a self-sustaining

organization, and instead of paying myself a salary, I opted to use the money I had raised to build a staff. Theresa, who had started as a volunteer, came on as our manager, working side by side with me and handling the mechanics of the organization. I also hired a farmer as our programs continued to grow. Requests for me to speak at events and mentor other patients became overwhelming, so with Theresa in charge, I escaped to the Boundary Waters Canoe Area (BWCA) with Ron and the girls to recover some much needed stamina. It was my favorite place to unplug, and I was anxious to get back out on the water and into the healing solitude of the wilderness.

August 2011
A few weeks before we were schedule to enter the BWCA, I tore my meniscus. I'm not kidding. I'm not even sure how, but my brother-in-law came to my rescue, repairing it and quickly getting me back on my feet. All I wanted was to disappear into the wilderness where no day was like another. My knee injury and weakened physical state presented a challenge on the portages, but I overcame it by fully appreciating the strength in my girls. They were superstars. Seven-year-old Hannah carried her own gear like a trooper, and EmmaGrace emerged as the athlete I knew she was. As my 12-year-old paddling partner, she was killing it. At each new camp sight, we worked together to set up the tarp, tents, and collected fire wood before swimming, telling stories, resting in hammocks, writing in journals, or reading books while soaking up the healing energy of the pines covering the terrain. By the fire, Hannah skillfully carved spears out of sticks to fend off any approaching bears and on stormy nights we sang together under the tarp. It was a little piece of heaven on earth for sure.

Almost every day we broke camp and portaged heavy packs across rugged trails, then navigated through lakes in search of our next campsite. By the third day, after a fairly long portage, we put our boats in at Temperance Lake and began our pursuit. Finding no empty sites, we strapped our packs to our backs and traversed another two miles, scrambling up a muddy trail to Cherokee Lake. By the time we found an empty camp site, we had covered 10 miles, which for most would have been a very difficult day, but my girls seemed no worse for the wear. Twice, Hannah had tripped, falling just out of reach in front of me. As she lay on the trail like a turtle on its back unable to right herself, I brought forth the strength of a mother and grabbed the handle of her back pack and pulled her uyp, setting her back on her feet in one sweeping motion. She wasted no time brushing off and much like the Ever Ready Bunny continued the march towards the water's edge.

Meanwhile Emma Grace, who never thought of herself as athletic, chewed up trail as she led the way to the next lake. When she arrived, she blew a long shrill on her orange safety whistle, encouraging us on. That sound never failed to give me the inspiration I needed to pick up the pace over those steep, deeply rutted trails, which were often slippery with moss covered roots and rocks or pocked with puddles as small rivers ran through them. Rarely did we find a trail that was easy to negotiate under the weight of our packs. Ron's job was to bring up the rear, carrying one canoe at a time. First he brought ours, giving us time to load it and push off shore while he went back for his own solo canoe.

Disappointed by the only camp left on Cherokee Lake, we hoped for something better the next day. What we had was a steep climb from the water, thickly wooded and over run by bugs. The pit toilet was a trick to get to, and if a bear did decide to pay us a visit, there was nowhere for us to go. I hardly slept and was grateful for the morning light. We were boiling water on the refreshed fire when Ron noticed a group leaving the island campsite an eighth of a mile across the water from us. It was too good of a site to miss. We scrambled to pack up two of our packs, throwing them in the boat for EmmaGrace and Ron to paddle over and quickly claim our new spot. It was a busy season in the BWCA, and good campsites were difficult to find. Ron placed our packs out in the open, so other canoeists wouldn't waste their energy paddling to the claimed site then left EmmaGrace to explore. Meanwhile, Hannah and I packed up the rest of our gear, loaded it into our canoe and paddled out into the sunshine excited to see the new site. We settled in on the island and vowed to stay for as many days as we could. It was the perfect place to play, perched on a massive rock left by the glaciers. Where it met the water on one side a shallow bay had formed, creating a lovely little spot for Hannah to swim. On the back side it rose high above a deep spot in the water, enticing Ron and EmmaGrace to enjoy an afternoon of cliff jumping while I played with Hannah in her lagoon. The days on Cherokee Lake were unequivocally the best days I had ever had with my girls. I laughed with absolute joy as they sang Lady Gaga to the passing loons who bobbed their heads to the beat, made egg cookies because cooking over the fire was more of a challenge than they had thought, watched frogs jump off cliffs into the water, painted themselves with mud to look like French men, made up silly jokes and were entirely without fear of bears or other night time critters. It was true serenity.

Every party has a pooper, and without a doubt I was it. I just couldn't seem to stay out of trouble. While changing into my swimming suit, I sprained my ankle. That's right. I was balancing on one leg, got dizzy and my ankle collapsed. I lay there crumpled with my bare butt on the ground and cried. Scooping me up from the dirt, my family worked hard to hold back their laughter while I pulled my bathing suit bottoms up and inspected the bruises forming quickly on my hip, butt and ankle. Simultaneously, my ankle ballooned into a flesh colored tennis ball attached to the base of my fibula, placing me firmly on hammock rest until the following day. I swaddled my ankle in a compression wrap and made room for Hannah to climb in for a snuggle while I read *Three Billy Goats Gruff* and *Flat Stanley*. I missed Emma Grace who was listening from her hammock, and reached out for her hand, wishing she was still small enough to climb in with us. My heart melted when she grabbed hold.

The Boundary Waters was a magical place where I loved to breathe the crisp northwoods air, touch the cool clear water and experience the earthy smells of the forest without any type of civilized interference. It was rejuvenating through and through. On our next visit a couple of years later, we arrived at the canoe launch in an unrelenting drizzle. Hanging around the launch was a group of Russian fathers and sons who had just come out from a week-long trip. Their gear was scattered throughout the launch site, forcing us to maneuver around and through their random piles to put our canoes in the water. Our spirits were already dampened by the rain, and their mess didn't help. We loaded our gear into the canoes while the Russians formed a circle. Holding hands, they released from their souls the most beautifully harmonized choral music we had ever heard. Amazed, I couldn't help but feel as if I was in a Disney movie. You know, the ones where something happens and you say to yourself, "that would never happen in real life." With our spirits lifted by their gift, we pushed off shore and waved good bye, thanking them as our boats glided smoothly through the calm lake waters.

April 2012
With staff picking up the slack at NuGenesis, I turned my attention to spending more time at home inventing or tweaking existing recipes. I stuffed green peppers with brown rice, pasture raised beef, Swiss chard, kale, onions, garlic, carrots and celery with Emmentaler and cheddar cheese. I made soup, using three different types of squash along with thyme, parsley, sage and rosemary. It was such a hit that my college-aged niece asked for her own jar as a Christmas present. After each growing season, I preserved tomatoes by cutting the small core off the end, plopping them in a zip-lock bag and tossing them in our chest freezer to be used another day. In that way, I could have farm-grown, organic tomatoes all year-round. When I was ready to use them, all I had to do was pull a tomato out of the bag, run it under warm water and slide the skin right off. In addition to quickly made spaghetti or pizza sauce, I made wonderfully fresh tasting salsa and basked in delight as I watched my kids gobble it up by the spoonful before asking for more.

August 2012
As our fruitful growing season drew-to-a-close, I took notice of a change in the skin on my reconstructed breast. It had become almost translucent, which was obviously not right, so I called Dr. Sanders. Since he had no available appointments, I had to meet his partner instead.

After scrutinizing my right breast, Dr. Kasdorf leaned back against the cupboards in the exam room and pompously reported, "The radiated skin is thinning. It won't be long before it tears open exposing the implant. I'm going to have to do a DIEP flap surgery, which you should've had from the start. I'll take healthy skin from your abdomen and use it to replace the failing skin on your reconstructed breast. You'll be happy with the results because you'll have a much more natural looking breast."

I was stunned by his arrogance along with the content of what he had said. It had never occurred to me nor had it ever been discussed that it was a possibility for my skin to fail. Having a plethora of complications already under my belt, you'd think I would've just rolled with it, but his description of what was to come filled me with dread. I discussed that same intricate surgery with Dr. Sanders before my mastectomy back in 2006, however, he had refused to offer it to me as an option. He had attended a plastic surgeon's conference where two female doctors on the panel admitted that they would never submit to the DIEP flap (Deep Inferior Epigastric Artery Perforator) surgery. Back in 2006 while I was preparing for reconstructive surgery, the DIEP flap was not favored over implants, but just six years later, it had become more common, and Dr. Sanders was on board with Dr. Kasdorf.

I had worked so hard to break free from medical protocols, but they just weren't willing to break free from me. Since my body grappled with recovering from anesthesia more and more, I needed to prepare it differently to withstand another brutal slice and dice. For that job I enlisted the help of Dr. David Rakel, the founder and director of the integrative medicine program at the University of Wisconsin Research Center. While he was one more doctor on my team of doctors, his skills were different than any of the others. He started with my heart, believing that it just needed a little help to repair itself and Coreg was holding it back. He first suggested I drop Coreg, replacing it with high doses of CoQ10 to improve my heart's function, and he was right. A later echocardiogram revealed a little step up in my EFR from 51% to 53%. Under Dr. Rakel's counsel I added resveratrol, vitamin C and vitamin B-complex to boost my immune system, a regimen he suggested I stay on for a full five weeks following surgery to help speed my recovery, which would take much longer than I was used to.

Finally, Dr. Rakel inquired, "How's NuGenesis going? Are you feeling at all stressed over it?"

I laughed uncomfortably before answering, "Yes. It's like a weight around my neck. I feel bad for saying that though. I made a commitment and feel as if I need to see it through even though my meditations seem to tell me otherwise.

225

I'm proud of what I've done, but it's just taking from me more than I'm willing to give."

"Well, that's something to think about," he said in a questioning tone.

He was right. I clearly had one very important task to complete before the impending surgical trauma. At the next NuGenesis board meeting, I broke the news that I could no longer work as executive director, CEO and development director, and it felt good. I decided to stay on the board but wouldn't be working in any other capacity for the organization. I prepared the staff for my departure, and when December arrived, I took my leave. I can't even describe how liberating it was to not have to read emails, answer calls, put out fires, attend meetings and write grant proposals. "Demoting" myself to board member, meant I could take a leave from the organization and focus on healing myself at my own pace, something I hadn't done since its founding.

December 2012

The DIEP flap surgery took more than 6 hours to remove the radiated skin, replacing it with a very large piece of skin taken from my abdomen, grafting it in place and creating a breast mound in the process. The recovery was arduous, requiring a six-day stay in the hospital, which felt like an eternity for me. I required continuous pain killers delivered through an epidural needle in my spine. Tubes came out of every part of my body, and there were more drain grenades than I could possibly count. The first night of recovery I spent in ICU with nurses checking the grafted tissue each and every hour looking for any sign of infection or tissue die off due to lack of blood supply. The second day, I was wheeled to the maternity ward where Dr. Kasdorf preferred his patients to recover. There were fewer babies that time of year, less scuttle butt on the floor and the nurses could focus most of their attention on my needs. While much of my time in that hospital room has been erased from my memory, there were some exceptions. Every day all day, my mom faithfully held vigil on the couch across from my bed. Whenever I opened my eyes, she was there, giving me the comfort only she could give. I couldn't begin to express my love for her and was deeply blessed by her presence.

Every morning at 6:00 a.m., Dr. Kasdorf appeared at my bedside to check my bandages. The first morning he appeared seemed like a dream. It was dark in my room, but a man wearing a trench coat and bolero was backlit by the street lights outside my window. I must've had a brief out of body experience because I watched from across the room as he bent over my sleeping body. At first I didn't realize it was him and was curiously alarmed before realizing it was my doctor gently lifting the myriad bandages to check my skin.

When I returned to my body and opened my eyes slightly, he gently said, "It's Dr. Kasdorf."

I closed my eyes and went back to viewing from across the room, and as quickly as he appeared, he was gone.

My family visited every day, sometimes to see me and more often to keep my mom company. I slept through the majority of that week, waking only when the nurses required me to get cleaned up or try to walk on my own. It felt as if my whole system had shut down and every ounce of energy I had was rushed to the massive surgical wounds stapled together across my torso. The pathology on the removed tissue identified "degenerated blood cells and rare inflammatory cells but "no malignant cells," and that was all that mattered. As I prepared to go home I reflected back on well-wishers' comments about how great it would be to get a tummy tuck out of the deal. If they had only known that four years later I would still be addressing complications from the DIEP flap, they might have just left it at wishing me luck.

During my recovery, Hannah often shared her profound thoughts brightening my mood.

On one occasion, she said, "You know, Mom, they say sticks and stones may break my bones, but words can never hurt me, but that's not true. Words scar your heart."

On another day at dinner, she broke out into a song by The Band Perry singing, "If I die young, bury me in satin." Then she paused and said, "But, Mom, if I die young, just bury me in my grubbies."

"Why your grubbies?" I asked.

She was very practical and responded with, "If I die, they're only clothes and I won't need them anyway."

Those kinds of moments reminded me of what I was missing by being away from my girls while working on NuGenesis and emboldened my decision to move forward and phase myself out. The first step to relinquish the president's role was already done. However, I was aware that divesting entirely might send the wrong message to our supporters who could think I was abandoning the ship all together, something I didn't want to happen. The organization was cruising along just fine with nine contracted dietitians, a couple of contracted educators, a farmer and a community outreach coordinator all supported by 100s of volunteers. Our work was being integrated into the programs at a

227

variety of hospitals in the area along with being used by corporations, schools and a variety of other community institutions. We were doing a ton of good, so I had to be careful.

February 2013

The month of February ushered in DIEP flap complications starting with a tear in my chest muscle under the flap. Somehow, not clearly explained to me, the tear created a blood filled seroma that quickly grew to the size of a grapefruit, sending me for the 700,090th time to the emergency room. The ER doctor called in the radiologist on duty to do an ultrasound on my chest, which confirmed that a fluid filled sack had formed. Radiologist Dr. Goran, another doctor I had never met, was called in to drain it. Much to my surprise he refused, reasoning that it was too complicated of a case. Oh boy, he wasn't kidding. I had lived it for seven plus years and all he was being asked to do was spend 30 minutes sucking out body fluid.

"Hang on. Don't leave yet. I'm going to call Dr. Doering," I said reassuringly to him, thinking if I wasn't panicked, maybe he wouldn't be either.

I called Dr. Doering on his cell phone who then spoke with the apprehensive radiologist, but to no avail. Dr. Goran held firm to his refusal, recusing himself for fear that if it was cancer he could do more harm than a good. Dr. Doering assured him that it wasn't cancer and that I was just highly unlucky. Even so, I respected Dr. Goran's decision, primarily because he was a rare breed of doctor who knew his limits, however, my emotions were sucked into another whirlpool of despair.

The following day found me in Dr. Kasdorf's procedure room, propped up on the exam table, waiting for him to arrive. When he walked through the door carrying a stainless-steel tray adorned with a large gauge needle, a pile of white gauze and a plastic bucket, he greeted me wryly. His deep disappointment was palpable and directed entirely at me. He was disappointed that "my" seroma had destroyed "his" perfect breast. He actually said something along the lines of "the breast I created was no longer pretty," making it clear that I had really let him down. I should've jumped off the table and bolted for my car since he was obviously devoid of compassion. Instead like a broken record, I took my poison as he aggressively jabbed the needle over and over into the mass, sucking out bloody fluid and draining the syringe in the sink. Dr. Kasdorf neglected to use an ultrasound which would've helped guide his moves, instead opting to blindly thrust the needle into my body repeatedly until he connected with my chest muscle. I screamed out in pain, which was met with his further disappointment and conclusion of his work. When I got home, I discovered the area was already heavily bruised and even more swollen than before.

A few days later, I went back to Dr. Kerrigan who agreed it needed to be drained, adding that she would not send me back to "Dr. Deranged." I waited in a chair while the technician prepared for the procedure and realized I could easily rest my chin on the expanded seroma, which oddly enough I found humorous.

"All set. Do you want to come over and lie on the table? Dr. Kerrigan will be in shortly," the technician asked rhetorically.

"No. I'd rather not," I responded half-joking.

I acquiesced and as soon as my back side hit the table, my blood pressure shot through the roof. I had forgotten to center my energy. Beads of sweat formed on my face before the good doctor even touched me. When Dr. Kerrigan arrived by my side with a kind smile, she picked up a tiny little needle attached to a syringe filled with Lidocaine and proceeded to inject the pain killer to deaden my nerves. Her next tool was a huge steel tube technically called a needle. She wasn't messing around. If there were blood clots in the seroma, they were going to be pulled out as well. As she breached my skin, I felt the pressure but no pain. Dr. Kerrigan used an ultrasound to guide her movements, and I watched the needle move through the scar tissue, bouncing like a car going over speed bumps. She continued to insert the needle into each pocket of blood scattered throughout my reconstructed breast. Through my ear phones the music of Native American flutist Kevin Locke calmed me down as I worked hard to transport myself to a place of peace. The whole ordeal lasted about 20 minutes and ended just as I was fighting my tongue not to yell, "STOP!" In total, Dr. Kerrigan removed five and one half large syringes of fluid, all of which she sent to the lab to have screened for cancer cells instead of dumping them down the sink drain as Dr. Kasdorf had.

She wrapped my chest in a compression bandage to help reduce future swelling, and before Dr. Kerrigan left the room, she commented, "I don't often see that result after a DIEP flap surgery."

I gave her a sad snicker and said, "I get it all."

Slightly disoriented, I slowly walked to the parking garage towards my car, trying to hold back the tears. All I wanted was to feel normal, which didn't seem as if it was too much to ask for. Once in my car, Ron called to see how it went and I broke down bawling and unable to speak. After a minute of unbridled sobbing and no conversation, I finally hung up. In the end, that seroma was drained four more times before Dr. Doering and Dr. Kerrigan recommended it be surgically removed by Dr. Kasdorf because "he was the only one who knew exactly where the blood supply was."

May 2013

Out of nowhere or perhaps not, Hannah asked if she could lead me in a guided meditation, directing me to a chair on the screened in porch then asking me to close my eyes. As I sat there she invited me to think of a place where I felt at peace. Now remember, she's only 10 years old and had never taken part in guided meditation.

"Now, tell me where you are," she commanded.

"I'm on a beach on the Pacific Ocean in the Olympic National Forest," I dutifully responded.

"That sounds pretty. I haven't been there yet," she said.

"Imagine your best fairy friend and a situation where you need your fairy's help, then tell me about it," Hannah commanded again.

"I'm in the mountains and I see a wolf that I want to pet, but my fairy stops me before it bites me," I recounted.

Hannah liked that story. Then I asked if we could just have a quiet meditation, to which she agreed, and I proceeded to pretend while she took a pile of my old business cards and laid them out on the floor to spell "We Are God's Love."

When we concluded our meditation session, Hannah asked, "Why do people limit themselves by saying the sky's the limit? It's not you know. They should say the Universe or Heaven is the limit."

"Yes, they should," I said.

One morning, I noticed that my bottles of daily supplements had grown way beyond what I had ever intended. I had vitamin D, fish oil, vitamin C, vitamin B complex, astragalus, echinacea, resveratrol, grape seed extract, turmeric, garlic, milk thistle, dandelion root, rhodiola, etc., and still, I wasn't feeling like a million bucks. Ruminating on how I had gotten there, I remembered countless internet searches and first hand recommendations leading me to mindlessly add supplements for one reason or another. Clearly, I had temporarily forgotten what I already knew – whole foods were always a better source of nutrients than supplements. In truth, most supplements were just a waste of time and money, parsing out the favored compounds from the whole food. However, there were always exceptions to that rule. If your body needs support for a specific reason, supplements could serve the purpose as in boosting the immune system. However, once the job was done, it was best to go back to the real deal. I used milk thistle and dandelion root to help recover my liver and milk thistle with dandelion leaves to help my kidneys return to normal function. Regrettably, I continued to spend unnecessary money on those two supplements even after my organs had healed.

In contrast to supplements, the nutritional components of whole organic foods were much easier for my body to absorb. When I chewed and swallowed food, the enzymes in my body set off a reaction, which was far more beneficial than taking one single component at a time. For example, doctors used to recommended that those taking vitamin E supplements were less likely to suffer from heart disease, but as the research deepened, it became clear that those taking vitamin E supplements actually increased their mortality rate. However those getting their vitamin E from whole foods such as nuts, seeds, whole grains, fish and leafy greens, suffered no adverse health effects. Then, there was always the high cost of the supplements to consider over the high cost of organic whole foods. When I did the math, I discovered that it was always cheaper for me to eat the real deal than to buy a piece of it in a bottle.

I did make a few exceptions to my daily supplement intake. For example, I used vitamin D and fish oil, which were both proven to provide significant benefits without the risks. Over the previous years, my triglyceride levels had climbed in part due to chemotherapy but also due to a genetic condition in my family. I took fish oil because it had serious science behind it showing that it could help improve cholesterol. In addition, fish oil had powerful anti-inflammatory properties, and I believed that for me, it was worth the cost. Vitamin D became another one of my staples, which was bolstered by recent studies linking higher levels of vitamin D to a reduction in cancer risk. Natural sources of vitamin D could be found in mushrooms, salmon, shellfish, eggs, cheese and the wonderfully rejuvenating sun, but in the event that I didn't get enough each day, I took the supplement as assurance.

June 2013
The time had come for me to prepare for having the persistent seroma removed, which meant I was called in for another MRI to identify exactly where it was. The scan identified a "5"x 4" 2"x 3" "loculated seroma." By that time, it was causing pain and regular muscle spasms in my neck and shoulder along with severe itching under the skin, and if you looked at me straight on, it was clear there was a significant difference in size between the two sides. Informed by the MRI, Dr. Kasdorf took me into surgery one more time. Afterwards, while I

231

slept off the anesthesia, he reported to Ron and my mom that he had removed nothing.

"I couldn't feel the seroma," he said.

Adding insult to injury, Dr. Kasdorf continued, "To help her muscle spasms, I was planning to balance the right side with the left by removing the extra fat I had placed during the DIEP flap, but I decided against it. If it really bothers her, I can go back in at a later date."

When my mom recounted his assessment to me, I was stunned. It was insanity that he so carelessly subjected me to another procedure under anesthesia and then did absolutely nothing of value. The seroma was clearly identified by the MRI, but he couldn't "feel" it? Dr. Kasdorf's nurse gave me my discharge papers, which listed that I was to call the office for a three month follow-up at which time he would decide whether I needed another surgery. I tossed those instructions in the garbage before leaving my room, declaring that he would never touch me again.

August 2013
Every day my body hurt. The muscles in my neck and around my collarbone were so painful that it became hard to turn my head. The scar tissue in my right reconstructed breast was itchy and the muscle spasms had gotten worse, causing me to struggle to do the simplest of tasks. My body in no way felt like my own, and reiki and meditation seemed to have met their match. I set up an appointment with one physical therapist after another, hoping to find someone that could untangle the mass of scarring under my skin, but it wasn't until I discovered Kathy Bussen that the final leg of my healing began. She was intelligent and hungry to learn. While she was semi-retired and only working part-time, Kathy continued to attend workshops and training to keep her skills current while at the same time exploring "alternative" techniques that might help her clients.

During our sessions, she described what she was doing in detail, teaching me how my anatomy worked and feeding my own abilities to self-heal. In the end, her skills helped to recover some of the hearing loss I had suffered from the parotidectomy, despite Dr. Harrison believing it was unrecoverable. However, it was a tough road. The radiated skin around the back of my left ear was thinning just like my breast tissue had, so Kathy had to work gingerly to loosen the scarring. Even so, she accidentally tore the skin, causing blood to ooze out and leaving her absolutely horrified and deeply apologetic. Everything she did to me caused pain and lots of it, but with her dedication month by month and year by year, progress was being made. Because of the mastectomy, I developed axillary web syndrome or cording, which meant the connective tissue in my chest, back and arm had hardened. Along with the scarring, cording caused extensive pain, restricting the range of motion in my arm and distorting the shape of my reconstructed breast. After four years of untangling that rat's nest, I was maybe 85% percent of the way back to almost normal, which was a huge gain. When Kathy first started working on me, she felt daunted by the amount of scarring I had but resolved to working on it as if she was peeling an onion. She was fearless in stretching and separating the painful tissue and unrelenting when it came to learning new techniques that might help me recover even faster. She left me in tears as she tackled the cording and scarring that twisted my rib cage out of alignment, and without exception each session left me exhausted, but I endured because little by little I felt my skeleton pull free from its painful anchor.

I couldn't help but think that if I had started with her immediately after my first surgery, the scarring wouldn't have been so extensive. Even today, surgeons are reluctant to recognize the post-surgical benefits of physical therapy for cancer patients. In 2017, Kathy's work with me was almost done and I couldn't have been more grateful. It had taken her more than four years to free my body, but it could've happened a lot faster had my insurance company allowed for more than 20 visits per year. The delay between the 20th visit and the new year resulted in the loosened scar tissue tightening again, setting my recovery back a few months. If they had allowed as many sessions as was necessary to complete the job, I might have finished within that first year.

As I continued to experience little shifts in my evolution towards transformation, what once caused me great anxiety, became a source of real hope. Each blood draw from my scarred veins, brought good news. My kidney numbers were improving and my liver numbers looked great. However, my intestines remained just as stubborn as their host. So ignoring the doctors that told me my intestines would never recover, I continued to work with Dr. Rakel to prove them wrong, remaining hopeful that some smart research scientist would find a way, or I would harness the healing power of my body to finish the job.

We made a celebratory trip to Washington Island, during which we embraced my improving physical state with bike rides throughout the Island's hilly terrain. We took the ferry over to Rock Island as we usually did, but on that trip we actually hiked to the light house and back, something I hadn't been able to do while in treatment. I wouldn't say it was easy for me, but I made it. Afterwards, we played on the beach and swam in the shallow, crystal clear, Caribbean blue waters of the bay at the end of the Havamal Trail. We enjoyed the tiny farmer's market where we discovered that we preferred purchasing food someone else grew instead of growing it ourselves.

Once home, we collected our tools from the barn and carried them out to the garden where we found an explosion of weeds assisted by the heavy rains that fell while we were away. I stood staring down at the rows, and knew I wasn't up for the task. The physical work of gardening caused my chest and arm to swell, mercilessly reminding me that I was not normal and may never be. Having been choked out by weeds, many of the plants had become stunted in the short time we were away, and even though I knew they were recoverable, I didn't want to be the one to do it.

"I just can't do it," I said.

"I don't want to either. It's a never-ending task, and you know how much I hate repetition," Ron replied.

"So that's it?" I asked.

"That's it," he said.

After harvesting what we could, we made the difficult decision to let our garden go. We maintained the fruit and asparagus beds for the following seasons then tilled the choked out beds before planting them back into pasture grasses. In October, we would turn the entire garden over to the horses who would prune the raspberry vines in preparation for the next year's crop. Our decision marked another step in my transformation, and for the rest of the season we supported our local organic farmers.

September 2013
Kid Rock performed in Milwaukee as part of his Harley-Davidson sponsored tour, and Ron's cousin Bill Davidson invited us to go. I was a little reluctant because I could barely stay awake past 9:00 p.m., but on the other hand, I didn't want to miss out on doing something a normal adult would do. So, I threw caution to the wind and embraced the event. At the venue we met up with Bill who escorted us to Kid Rock's back stage room where the rest of the group was milling around. I stood off to the side, trying to block out the overwhelming noise in that tiny space and reserve my energy for the show. We watched from the side stage, dancing and cheering for the entire energized concert. I often lost my balance but generally caught myself before crashing to the ground in hysterics.

The after party was low key and kind of sad. Kid Rock was buried in the middle of his small entourage not talking to any of his fans. After a great concert, it was fun to tell the band how much you loved the show and snap a picture for memories, but that was a no go with The Kid. Each of us was instructed that there were to be no pictures and no one was to approach him to talk. Basically, we were supposed to act as if he wasn't even there. Our group sat on the couches chatting when Bob, Kid Rock, took us by surprise and sat down next to me. He started to chat as if we had known each other for some time and struck me as the typical Midwest boy who happened to hit it big as a rocker.

"Did you watch the show?" he asked through a pursed-lip smile.

"It was a great show tonight! I saw you play at the 100th Harley-Davidson anniversary as well and loved your political satire. You know being here makes me look kind of cool to my 15-year-old daughter. So thanks for that," I said laughing at myself.

"Oh! Happy to," he replied looking at me as if he was waiting for me to say something else.

Not to disappoint, I added, "This was the first concert I've been to since recovering from cancer."

Once it was out I wanted to take it back, but he acted as if he already knew.

"My sister had cancer but is doing okay now. My dad has it too and he's not doing so well," Bob shared as he looked down at his hands.

 "I'm so sorry. Cancer really sucks. There's just so much of it out there," I continued, understanding that cancer was the true equalizer.

Clearly feeling bolstered by my comment, Bob said a toast to his dad followed by, "Fuck cancer. I think I'll write that song. It's the name of an organization in Canada. Do you think that's OK?"

"Why not?" I responded.

I wished his dad well, then Bob introduced me to his girlfriend before burying himself back in his small entourage. Ron laughed at the odd exchange, but sometimes things happen for a reason. In that case, whatever it was, it was clearly for Bob. He needed to say what he said and had decided I was the person he was going to say it to.

October 2013
The wonderfully cool fall days lit a new source of energy inside me with

mindfulness at its core. I loved to practice, taking in as many details as I could from where ever I was and what ever was happening around or inside me. It was the brightest silver lining of the many bestowed upon me during my cancer battle and awakened me to who I was and what I was meant to do. Mindfulness also helped me recognize that cancer was not as evil as it had first appeared. During my battle, I learned to stop and listen, open fully to the peace in my faith and embrace the release of fear and worry. Cancer gave me a framework by which to make better choices in my life and balance my energy in a way that I could serve myself and others. Through it I garnered an understanding of the power I had within and how to tap my God given ability to self-heal. Finally, cancer helped me to understand that even with so much loss, there would always be peace. I'm not saying it was a wonderful experience to have cancer. I'm simply saying since I had it, I had to make the best of it, and I think I did.

I tested my recovering strength and evolved mindset on a trip to Arizona with Ron and a group of his running friends. Their plan was to run from the southern rim of the Grand Canyon to the northern rim and back to the southern all in one day. The 80-mile route was iconic among ultramarathon runners, and our group had been eagerly planning and training for nearly a year when a couple of days before the run, Ted Cruz decided a government shutdown was exactly what the people of America needed in order to see things his way. Among other things, he closed all of the parks to the very public who were paying for them.

Making lemonade out of lemons, some of the runners headed to Flagstaff while others ran through the desert around Sedona. Ron and I did both, staying in Sedona for a couple of days before driving up to Flagstaff where we met two other couples. There, we hiked nearby Humphrey's Peak, the tallest mountain in the area. While in treatment I would've been terrified to attempt such a hike, but those feelings were long gone. I embraced what I thought would be a peaceful day hike in the wilderness but found it to be anything but. When we arrived in the parking lot at the base of the mountain, it was full of cars that would have otherwise been at the Grand Canyon, and outdoor enthusiasts overran the trail because there was nowhere else for them to go. We joined the precession, and step by step I deliberately navigated the rugged trail as Ron dawdled with his hands cupped behind his back in boredom. He walked that way for almost five miles, and while I felt a twinge of guilt for holding him up, I brushed it off, knowing that he was fully aware of my limitations. I stayed focused on each step, pausing to breathe whenever I felt dizzy, and while I couldn't be fast, I was steadily moving towards the peak rising 12,000 feet above sea level. I found myself questioning whether I would make it before realizing that the more important question was did I really care.

At a little over four miles, Ron gingerly suggested that I might not be able to make it to the peak, and even though I thought he might be right, I was still hurt by his desire to quit on me. I forced myself to mindfully take a reading of my body. My legs were shaking, and I grew dizzier the higher we got. I lost my balance more often and was creating a bottle neck for the crowds of people trying to move past me as they trudged their way to the summit.

I began a dialogue with myself, "I don't need to summit. I'm not enjoying the hike as I might've, if the trail had been primarily empty. Maybe Ron's right. Maybe I shouldn't push myself to the point where I get hurt."

When we reached the turn to traverse the last 600 feet of trail, I studied the path leading to the peak. It was covered in shale rock and our fellow-tourists looked like a line of ants marching to the queen. I envisioned tripping on people or rocks as I carefully maneuvered my way up. It wasn't the type of wilderness I enjoyed. Instead, I preferred solitude, and I wasn't as goal focused as the rest of our group. My hike that day was about challenging myself and I had done that. So at 11,400 feet, I stopped. I knew Ron would continue to walk up with me if I wanted to, but I didn't want to. I stepped off the trail and waved him on to complete his goal. After I peeled off, I watched him take one sluggish step, wait, take another and wait. It was clear that he wouldn't be down for some time. He was locked into the line of tightly packed vacationers traipsing their way up the rocky single track trail to Humphrey's Peak. Grateful for the day, I found a sunny spot in view of the trail and rested. I chatted with people as they waited to move one more stride, feeling a slight desire to jump in step. It was the shadow of my old self popping up, and as quickly as she appeared, she disappeared like vapor. I wasn't that person anymore, and an older gentleman I had never met stopped, faced me and smiled.

He stepped out of line and asked, "Are you enjoying the sunshine?"

With a wide grin, I answered, "Yes, I am."

Then, out of nowhere he asked, "Did you have cancer?"

"Yes. Why do you ask?" I questioned him.

"My sister did too. I'm a retired doctor. Why aren't you going to the summit?" he asked continuing his inquiry.

"I don't need to. I'm happy with my hike today. Maybe I will another time," I said with a shrug.

"That's exactly what my sister would say. Enjoy your time and don't let anyone push you to do something you don't want to do. It was so very nice to meet you," he said with deep sincerity as he stepped back on to the trail.

That little exchange was the happiest moment of the entire trip. Instead of waiting for Ron to walk me back down and still grinning from my exchange with the retired doctor, I nudged my way against the crowd and moved back down the mountain. I knew Ron would catch up with me some time later, and when he did, he gushed about the spectacular views but lamented the crowds. Since he had done what he had gone there to do, his demeanor was much more relaxed. Joel and Sandee, one of the couples in our group, flew past us as they raced down.

"I can't believe how far you made it without any training," Joel said as he continued moving.

He meant it to sound like praise, but I felt oddly offended and wanted Ron to tell him what I used to be capable of, but he didn't say a word. So, I did.

"I'm deceptively strong and resilient. Slow and steady wins the race!" I called as he skipped down the switchbacks.

November 2013
With winter approaching, I grew introspective about our time on the farm. While I was grateful for it, I was also growing tired of it. There was always work to be done whether it was feeding chickens and horses, cleaning the coop and stalls, or fixing out buildings battered by the weather. The chores were endless, and I was tired. The one thing I could say was that it was never dull, which couldn't have been demonstrated any better than it was on the morning of November 7. I woke up at 6:45 a.m. to the fearful and ferocious barks of our dogs. I cracked the window and as my groggy hearing tuned in, I heard what sounded like a truck driving on our gravel driveway, leaving me to wonder why the dogs were so uncharacteristically upset. Outside, I could hear my family chattering as they got into the car, but instead of driving down the driveway to go to school and work, they drove up to the barn.

I made my way downstairs to check out the commotion, and when I opened the door, Hannah exclaimed, "It's cows! Look at the cows, Mommy!"

I realized the sound on the gravel driveway wasn't tires at all, it was hooves. I grabbed the dogs and brought them in from the morning darkness, then went back out onto the deck where I could just make out the silhouette of a small herd of cattle back lit by the barn light. Ron had driven the girls up to see them and I could hear EmmaGrace laughing hysterically. She loved animals and the

238

excitement of something new and different caused her to launch out of the jeep and run towards the herd. In an instant, my amazement turned to terror at the thought of her fragile little body being trampled by the disoriented cows. I ran towards her yelling for her to stop when I noticed several other cows in the yard. I snatched EmmaGrace and Ron used the jeep to slowly push the stragglers away from us and move them through the yard to rejoin their herd. There were 22 in all and we had no idea where they came from. Since I was better with the animals, we agreed that Ron would take the girls to school while I tried to find out whose cows we were harboring. After several calls, I surmised we had Arnie Korth's little herd, or rather his daughter's. Arnie had recently passed away, and his kids were managing or more accurately, mismanaging the herd. It was the second time those cows had escaped, and it was our lucky day to have them visit us after a morning of crashing over the river and through the woods. I caught Arnie's son Craig on the phone and within a few minutes, he joined me in the barnyard. He was somewhere in his 20's and when he got out of the car, he stood staring at the cows, saying nothing to me.

"Are they yours?" I asked.

"Yeah, they're ours. They ran through a bunch of gates this morning and then crossed the highway," Craig reported.

After crossing the highway, I learned the herd had disappeared into the woods before materializing at the end of our driveway seeking refuge.

"Well, what do you want to do?" I asked confused.

He looked at me with a blank stare and said, "Well, my sister will be home from work around noon, so we'll figure it out then."

"Wait a minute," I said. "You can't just leave them here to wander around destroying our gardens and yard."

He met my eyes with an innocent ignorance, making it clear that he didn't have the slightest clue what to do. Without hesitation, my old self sprang into action. I directed him to pick up the metal fence panels leaning against the barn. I pointed to where I wanted him to place each panel as we built a pen to contain the herd. He moved quickly, following my lead to create a chute which would make it easier to control the cows as we moved them from the barnyard into the pen, hopefully removing any chance they would break free. I placed a few hay bales inside the round pen to entice the cows and gave Craig a crash course in the same herding techniques I had learned with Albert. It worked. Together, we moved the cows quietly and calmly into the pen under the watchful eyes of the horses.

When Craig turned to leave, he said, "I'll be back to pick them up a little later."

That was it. There was no expression of gratitude or humble apology for the trouble his cows had caused me, and even though he lived across the street from us, it took him two hours to return with a small two-cow trailer. For the rest of the afternoon, Craig arduously loaded his cows two by two, drove them home and then returned for the next pair. When it was all said and done, our gravel barnyard was destroyed along with the paddock where Craig had backed up the trailer 11 times throughout the day. I watched as he drove the last pair down the driveway and out onto the town road. I never saw him again.

The rest of the month, my schedule slowed substantially. The garden was closed down and we had put the food up for the winter. I was still speaking on behalf of NuGenesis but had no grants to write or staff to manage. I had no sick friends to care for, no dogs to train, no surgeries to prepare for or recover from, and I realized the only thing left to do was cook. I engrossed myself in developing my own techniques if you could call them that and honed my own creative flare. I made up recipes on the fly and truly enjoyed my time alone in the kitchen, creating art with each and every meal. My soups were big hits, and my vegetable medleys were devoured in record time. I added quinoa, barley, wheat berries and other whole grains to our menu along with the whole grain pasta and breads I had already been using. Our primary diet was complex carbohydrates with farm raised chickens or turkeys purchased from a local organic farmer. I perfected the roasted chicken, serving it with a side of quinoa and roasted vegetables. It was super easy, quick to prepare and always a hit. Sometimes, I slathered the chicken with kalonji oil, which added a surprisingly wonderful flavor despite its raw, rancid smell. The girls cleaned their plates, and I swelled with pride over my farm to table meals.

Hannah often joked about how I had become faster than Rachel Ray and her 30-minute meals, adding that mine were probably even healthier. We were always busy, running from one event to another and often not getting home until 7:30 p.m., but I always had time to cook something tasty. Sometimes, I was able to plan ahead and put a meal in the crock pot, but most other nights I threw a bunch of sautéed vegetables together with a whole grain or eggs, made grilled cheese and spinach on sprouted whole grain bread from a local bakery, or threw a pizza together, using premade sprouted whole grain dough from Angelic Bake House. I chopped veggies, opened a jar of my home-made pizza sauce, grated up some cheese and turned it over to the girls to literally throw what they wanted on top. Then, I popped it in the oven for 15 minutes – done.

240

Healthy, happy kids!

December 2013

During a follow-up echocardiogram, I was fortunate to have Jan as my technician. I had never met her, but she was instantly comfortable with me, opening up about how much her sister had changed since being diagnosed with cancer and how hard that was on her family.

"How are you so happy? I mean you seem so positive and happy. I want my sister to be that too," Jan confessed.

"I wish I could tell you I've found peace but that would be a lie. I have battled daily to push back at the fear, anger, frustration and uncertainty that two cancer diagnoses left me with. I've spent an inordinate amount of time searching for the silver linings and try to recognize that hosting cancer wasn't all bad," I responded doubtful I was helping her.

As Jan continued to perform the EKG, I drifted into my own reflections, training my mind's eye on the silver linings that had gotten me where I was. I was often asked how I did it and had to be honest. It wasn't easy. I had to dig deep to learn how to advocate for myself and get treatments I otherwise wouldn't have gotten. I had to dig even deeper to show up whether it was for treatment, for my family or for myself. Starting an organization to share what I had learned took my advocacy outside of myself and into the community, which led to my further evolution into someone who offered hope and strength to others. I had no idea if I would ever entirely transform into the person I was meant to be, but I was certain it was a continuous process of learning to live intentionally and without fear. If someone asked me what the secret of life was, I'd say to change everyday into someone better than I was the day before.

The last time I saw Dr. Rakel before he took a job in New Mexico, he explained how he believed I became cancer free, "There are three human characteristics shared by those who do well with cancer. They have a strong social support system, the ability to roll with the "punches," and they never take no for an answer. Kathy, you fit all three of those characteristics. Remember, that which we give attention to grows. There is no reason for you to doubt where you are today. You are simply proactive and were able to recognize the self-healing abilities in your body and then acted upon them. In my work, I've found that proactive patients always do better than passive ones."

I deeply valued his kind and very thoughtful words, but I didn't always "roll with the punches." It was hard not to give attention to the aggregate of side effects that made each day a little bit harder, but I heard his point loud and clear. I was deeply grateful for the caché of doctors I enjoyed who were willing to work on the same integrative medicine page as I was, supporting me in my desire to go beyond sanctioned protocols. How could I explain that to Jan? I did what I did because that was who I wanted to be. It was up to her sister to decide who she wanted to be. Some steps forward were easy for me but most were not. Telling her that change didn't come gracefully for me, may not have been at all helpful to her, and I didn't really know how my family felt about it, but from my perspective, change felt great.

January 2014
Another year, another New Year's pledge, and with sincere intentions, I proclaimed that 2014 would be my year of abundance, starting with bouncing belly laughs at John and Sheila's annual New Year's Eve party in Madison. It was a big crowd that year and at midnight we all laughed our way out onto the frozen lake in - 20° temperatures. About 50 yards from shore, we let out woops and cheers to ring in the New Year, then ran with teeth chattering back to the warmth of their cozy house. My official New Year's pledge was no surprise to anyone who knew me. I pledged to stay on the track that God had made for me and to scrutinize distractions while being aware of false paths.

Dr. Rakel once said to me, "There is no way to not be a different person after cancer than the person you were before it, because changing is inescapable after something so traumatic."

He was absolutely right.

I would hit 50 years old in 2014 and didn't think of myself as old, just more experienced. I had enjoyed so much in my life, traveling down so many different roads and trying to learn something from each and every one. In 2014, I carried no baggage forward. I carried no ill will or guilt. I left all expectations in 2013, pledging to experience pure love and joy, renewed health and vigor, and peace and abundance in whatever I did while accepting every event graciously and without judgment.

"Start at the present moment- accepting things exactly as they are – and search for my way in the midst of these circumstances." – Psalm 52:8 proverbs 3:5-6 AMP

Hello, 2014!

February 2014
"Be yourself, no matter how small and trust that the ultimate impact on the planet will be positive." Novelist Gail Godwin

242

The New Year brought a renewed ability to reconnect with individual patients through mentoring, starting with Tibisay. Within the first few seconds of our conversation, I felt drawn to her. Actually, it was more than that. I felt attached to her. Even though we had never met, Tibi confided in me, sharing her deepest emotions during our very first conversation. Over the next year, Tibi was a spot of sparkling light in my life. Her smile was direct from heaven. She was joyful, playful, loving, and comfortable on her path, in herself, and with her decisions. She was a lover of life, and her Nicaraguan energy was infectious. I had no doubt I had been blessed by her invitation to hang out in her space and felt a deep sense of joy in knowing Tibi and her willingness to know me. Our last meeting happened over breakfast in Madison, and Tibi was as radiant as ever. While we ate, she explained her decision to no longer submit to scans, tests or treatments.

"I'm happy. I feel great! I don't need to live in that world anymore," she explained with an aura of joy surrounding her.

I stared at her in awe, knowing that what she was really telling me was that she had decided to let her body die. She was vibrating at the highest level and it was time for her to go home.

"I can see you have no doubt about the decision you're making and I'm excited for you," I said spellbound by her spirit.

I was going to miss her, but I couldn't bring myself to say that out loud. Tibi insisted on paying for breakfast, and we embraced outside on the side walk. Before getting in my car, I watched as she skipped to hers, turned and waved good bye one last time, flashing her signature sun drenched smile. Just a few weeks later, I heard that she was gone. She had said her good byes and on a Monday was checked into the hospital with vertigo. Two days later, her body died. I called David, our shared reiki master, to let him know, and together we cried for our loss. Tibi was ready to take on the next phase of her work, and I felt so blessed to have been able to linger in her glow one last time.

After Tibi passed, I realized I hadn't evolved as far as I had thought. I became resistant to spending time with friends, but my resistance seemed to grow from an understanding that the more friends I had, the more friends I had with cancer and the more friends I had that died.

As New York talk show host Joe Franklin once said, "The average age of my friends is dead."

243

March 2014

The eve of St. Patrick's Day had arrived and while I had always loved decorating to celebrate our heritage, my limited energy stores left me to fall short with Hannah graciously picking up the baton. Incorporating green into every part of our day, Hannah made an elaborate leprechaun trap in her bedroom out of yarn and wove bells through every item in her room. When the leprechaun came to take her coins, she'd be able to hear him before he could escape. In the end her design proved to be less of an obstacle for the leprechaun and more of an obstacle for me. I usually slipped into the girls' rooms and took the pennies they had stacked on the floor, leaving behind chocolate coins scattered about, but with Hannah's new system, I couldn't get anywhere near her pennies. So, I waited for her to fall asleep and stood in the doorway of her room wondering what to do, and with no good options, I tossed the chocolate coins into the trap, letting them fall where they may and called it a night.

In the morning, Hannah came down dressed in every piece of green clothing she could find including the green hat headband I had bought for her at Walgreens.

She wrapped her arms around Skip, our Irish wolfhound, and said to me, "Top of the mornin' to ya!"

How could I resist her cheer? I pledged to make corned beef, made from locally grown cows raised on good, clean pasture, along with organic cabbage, potatoes and carrots. Just as my Irish mom had done.

On March 25, I turned 50. It was a great day to express my deep gratitude for my life, and I said a little prayer:

"Lord, there are so many good people struggling with chronic illness in my circle and beyond and so many struggling with cancer. Please show them the way to healing whether you are granting healing of the body, the spirit or both. Provide them with a strong support system and give them peace. If they have children, maybe you could let them beat cancer this time. As far as the children I know with cancer, I don't get your end game there. I just wonder if you're trying to create such outrage in our communities that we are all powerless to do anything other than stop the greed that hurts so many and benefits too few. If only it truly was a human right to breathe clean air, drink clean water and eat clean food. Now that cancer has become common, maybe your light will shine brighter on those profiting from our suffering and cause them to make much needed change. You know that the majority of the cancers we suffer could be prevented, so how about we make that happen now?"

My mom managed to wrangle my siblings and nephews together for a celebratory lunch on my behalf. I couldn't believe they were all there and was overwhelmed with appreciation. I knew it had to have been quite an effort for my mom to pull off, but her commitment to her kids was unmatched. In the evening, Ron and the girls took me to a French restaurant and proudly presented me with a beautiful pendant of malachite, pearl, sapphire, aquamarine and chrysocolla in a silver setting. Ron reminisced that it reminded him of the pearl earrings he had gotten me when we first started dating, the malachite necklace he had bought for me in Africa and aquamarine because it was my birthstone. I was deeply touched and once again grateful to be 50.

May 2014
Each morning on the screened in porch, I read *JESUS CALLING,* a gift from my mother-in-law. At first, I found it repetitive but came to realize that repetition was exactly what I needed to hone my practice in mindfulness. Before the girls made their groggy way downstairs, I took a few minutes to notice the tiniest of details. For example, the crabapple tree was in full bloom with pink-tinged white blossoms and the lavender-colored clusters of lilac flowers drenched the air with their sweet scent. The maples were always the first to fully leaf out, followed by the ginkgo then finally the black walnuts. The air was dense with moisture, gathering like small crystals dusting the screens on the porch. When the empty space between the wires became too burdened with water, strands of liquid irrigated a line of squares, streaking its way down to the ground. Most mornings, there was a multitude of birds flittering about from tree to tree, and I trained my ears to separate their unique songs. The red wing blackbird's bravado was dominant in the air, making it difficult to distinguish from the oriole, bluebird, indigo bunting, flicker or scarlet tanager. On the other hand, because their calls were well known to me, the sparrow, robin and chickadee stood out as soon as they joined the choir. Out on the prairie it seemed comfortably cool as the sun rose over my left shoulder, lighting up the golden marsh grass. I took a moment to send gratitude to the heavenly energy that provided my family with the divine blessing to restore that landscape back to a more natural state and to transform our old farm house into a thing of beauty.

By 7:00 a.m., the kids made their way down to the kitchen, and soon after, I heard Hannah complaining that EmmaGrace had taken all of the raspberries and blueberries, leaving her none for breakfast. Ahh, every cell in my body smiled. My kids were arguing over fruit. It truly was a perfect world. After they left for school, I returned to my solitude and engaged in mediation. At David's urging, I had received my reiki attunement for level one and opened further to embracing my practice of living in the moment and being open to all that was placed in my path. I focused my meditations on feelings of deeper peace and

245

opening to the spiritual connection I had been born with.

July 2014

To continue the healing of my little family who had suffered right along with me, Ron and I decided another adventure to Northern Minnesota for some unplugged play time with the girls was in order. Instead of the BWCA, we chose to explore the Isle Royale wilderness, which sat in Lake Superior off the coast of Minnesota. On the drive north, we noticed a sign advertising guided zip-line excursions through the canopy of the Boundary Waters. We looked at each other simultaneously and without saying a word agreed to turn off the highway and follow the signs along the gravel roads of northern Minnesota's backwoods seeking a new type of adventure.

"Why are we going this way? The island is the other way," EmmaGrace smartly asked.

"We're taking a little detour. Do you know what zip-lining is?" I asked.

"Of course we do," Hannah and EmmaGrace responded in unison.

"Well, Dad and I have decided we'd like to take a little detour and go zip-lining through the canopy of the Boundary Waters. We've never seen it from the top of the trees. Does that sound like fun?" I asked somewhat rhetorically.

"Yea!!!!" they cheered.

When we arrived at the resort, the sky grew thick with grey clouds moving quickly on the wind. While the shifting weather gave us a moment of pause, we threw caution to the wind, literally, and signed the waiver releasing the company from any and all injury we might sustain. Clearly other vacationers had displayed more common sense then we had, seeking shelter in the lodge and leaving us to sail through the canopy alone. The young guides Joe and Adam were assigned to our family. They dressed us in harnesses and heavy leather gloves to protect our hands, which would be our only breaks on the cable. We followed them around the back of the zip-line shed to a short expanse of cable just 15 feet off the ground. There, they quickly demonstrated the breaking technique and asked us to practice. After a few times of doing it correctly, we were directed to a waiting open air jeep.

Joe drove us up into the thickly vegetated hillside before stopping at the base of what looked like a short fire lookout tower. We climbed its stairs to a platform maybe 20 feet up, positioned ourselves, then leapt off, whizzing through a clearing in the canopy and landing on the next wooden deck wrapped around a massive tree some 30 yards away. Platform after platform we zipped through the trees, laughing at each other's technique and teasing about falling off the exposed landing pads as they swayed in the angry winds. We laughed until we hit the second to the last platform perched on top of a steep cliff. There was nowhere to go but off, and just as Joe was ready to lead the way, an unexpected thunder and lightning storm engulfed the skies above us dumping buckets of rain. We stared saucer-eyed at our guides who looked almost as worried as we were.

"Thanks to the storm, it's a race to the end. This is very dangerous to be out here, but we don't have a choice now. Remember, it's hard to break when the cable is wet, so start early. When you get to the other side, I'll be there to switch your safety line and get you off to the end. We're only two lines away from the safety of the shed, so let's get there quickly," Joe, the oldest of the two, sternly instructed.

Joe went first quickly followed by Ron and then EmmaGrace. Through relentless winds, the lightning seemed to be striking all around us, and with Hannah up next, she froze.

Adam looked at me and without reservation said, "You're going to have to throw her off."

Hannah clung to me, but I knew he was right.

I did my best to shelter her from the pelting rain as I took her little chin in my hand and said, "Honey, I don't want to do this, but I have to for you to be safe. We don't have time to be afraid. You have to go. Now, turn around."

Accepting her fate, Hannah whimpered, turned and terrified I pushed my baby off the cliff, watching in horror as she flew across the wet cable and slammed into the arms of Joe, waiting on the swaying platform at the other end. He sent her on to Ron, and then I vacated the cliff with my hands clasped tightly around the cable, trying to slow down before crashing into Joe.

Once my feet touched the platform, Joe ripped my safety line from one cable and slapped it on to the other yelling, "Go!"

I was shaking with fear by the time I touched down on the other end. Ron unclipped both safety lines and I looked up through the sheets of rain to thank God for keeping us safe. EmmaGrace watched from under the porch of the shed, laughing uncomfortably in disbelief. Hannah's tears slowed as we dragged our soggy bodies through the parking lot, absorbing the exhilaration of our adventure. While we stood at the car soaked to the bone, an uncontrollable emotional release took over and we all laughed so hard we had to race like four slapstick clowns to the bathroom.

September 2014
Prior to the cancer diagnosis, God mostly came into my thoughts when I had a problem or was worried. I think I could've been described as an "opportunistic worshiper." But over the course of my battle with cancer, I developed a desire, actually more like a need to connect every day and express gratitude for the blessings in my life. I asked God to help me live the life he intended for me and essentially begged for patience with my kids. Sometimes, I tried to picture God's face when I felt frustration well up from the depths, and while I did see Him a couple of times, it was his protective white light that mostly came through. In lieu of nothing at all, I learned to trust that I was still being heard and that sometimes there's nothing to do but wait. If I felt myself drowning in emotions, I reminded myself to sit quietly and ask for patience, trust, strength and healing as I waited in limbo for the answers to my prayers.

It would've been easy to wallow in that state of my weakened body with the persistent rib pain and constant buzzing in my head like cicadas droning away against my ear drums. Instead, I worked daily to remind myself to trust that every challenge was an opportunity to grow. Even so, it was relatively easy to veer off my path and bump into despair. My search for silver linings was endless until one day I found gold in the passage from *JESUS CALLING,* which described "God's gold tinged love of approval," and when I closed the book to think about that, the ginkgo tree outside the living room window blinded me with its glowing, gold-colored leaves. Back lit by the sun, its vibrancy almost hurt my eyes. I stood next to the window staring into its radiance and washed in the warmth emanating from its outstretched branches as it melted my discomfort away. It was at that moment that I realized I didn't need to search for God's approval, it was just exactly wherever I was.

October 2014
It had been 10 Halloweens since my diagnosis. Metaphorically speaking I had gone to the dark side, but on that 10th Halloween, I decided to literally go to the dark side. There was a haunted house farm called "The Darkside" near our house, which doubled as a petting zoo the rest of the year. During October weekends, the haunted farm thrilled all ages and earned the title of "Best Haunted House In Wisconsin" several years in a row. It was somewhat physically demanding, starting with a long and difficult to navigate descent into a recreated mine shaft, passing through its chambers of imprisoned ghouls and emptying out onto a spooky bonfire, where we waited for the hay wagon to collect us for a bumpy ride along a creepy wooded trail, crawling with ghosts

248

and goblins. It took a little more than an hour to make it to the end, but no one really wanted it to stop. It was funny, scary, creepy and exhilarating, and I loved every second of it. At the end of the wagon trail, we met Granny Nanny who, dressed like a wild-eyed woods woman, led us to a walking path that took us through the trees past a "toxic waste site" with monsters emerging out of the muck.

"Look, Mom! You don't look like any of them. I guess you're not the toxic avenger after all," EmmaGrace yelled through her laughter.

November 2014
Since Dr. Harper had retired in 2013, Dr. Doering sent me to see Oncologist Dr. Rafikki. My plan was not to go back to the cancer center ever again, but Dr. Doering wasn't comfortable with that, and even though I believed I was done with cancer, fear still lurked around the edges, so I agreed. I had no idea how hard it would be to step back into the cancer center once again. I wasn't sick. I didn't intend to get sick, and yet, I felt sick. A flood of old feelings washed over my body and my blood pressure rose as I once again sat in the chair for family members staring at the reclining treatment chair that was once meant for me.

When Dr. Rafikki walked into the room, I was pleasantly thrown off by her question, "So, why are you here?"

I explained that Dr. Doering had wanted an oncologist to keep eyes on me, which sent her to my chart. Dr. Rafikki flipped through the neatly organized pile of pages, talked about follow-up and after almost an hour, announced that there was no need for me to come back.

Concluding my appointment, Dr. Rafikki instructed, "I don't want you to have any scans other than the 3-D mammography. The normal CT scan equals 100 chest x-rays and we're likely to give you cancer all over again, if we keep exposing you. As far as recurrence goes, your left breast isn't out of the woods yet. It could have a primary diagnosis, which is why I want you to keep having mammograms. Other than that, you're free to go. Call me if you have any questions, fear, pain, something suspicious going on or a good restaurant recommendation."

And just like that, I was no longer a cancer patient.

March 25, 2015
My 51st birthday arrived, wrapping me in deep gratitude. It was an old practice among women to joke, lie, or even refuse to answer the question of age all together. I, on the other hand, embraced my age and as part of my

transformation decided to really "know myself." Several years earlier, during an activity in a support group session at Stillwaters, I was asked to list my character traits. I sat with that request for a moment before declining to participate. If I didn't want to share my deepest opinions of myself, I felt it wasn't fair for me to stay and listen to others expose theirs, so I went home. I don't know why I felt so uncomfortable. Maybe I was afraid of what I would discover during that tumultuous time, or maybe I didn't want anyone to really "know" me, including myself.

Approaching 10 years post diagnosis and after oodles of help moving towards the person I wanted to be, I no long carried those fears. So over a cup of coffee and my opened journal, I set my intention to be real and began writing. Some of what ended up on that page both surprised me and seemed obvious. I was alive and well. That was good. I was quiet and loud. Was that good? I was calm and excitable, and peaceful and agitated. I was lazy and motivated, humble and expectant, and gracious and needy. I was a caretaker, protector, leader and follower. I was loved and I loved deeply. I was grateful and resentful, and happy and sad. I was hopeful. I was open and very closed. I was a dreamer and a pragmatist. I was part of nature and disconnected. I was passive and aggressive. I was sensitive and harsh. I was a series of contradictions, forever working to sync my soul to the universal energy around me. I was still finding my way as I grew and changed. I left past wrongs in the past and was changed by cancer. I was a different person than when I was 20, 30 or even 40-years-old. I was better than I was and improving all the time. I was smarter, having learned that cancer was puny in our universal awesomeness. I was deeply grateful and forever humbled.

October 24, 2015
I completed another trip to Jackson Hole, Wyoming with Sheila to recognize the 10 years since my diagnosis, and neither one of us could process just how quickly that time had gone. While I was in the thick of it, the second hand of my watch moved laboriously. I reflected on the big differences between my ability to keep up between our first trip and the last, which was much more ambitious than any of the others. The first day, we hiked a nearly 10-mile route around Phelps Lake, which connected to a small bit of the Granite Canyon Trail leading back to our car. It was a thrilling day for me, and I'd like to think Sheila shared in that. I was able to keep up with her without any trouble and thoroughly enjoyed our lakeside lunch, overlooking the crystal clear water of Phelps Lake. Overhead, the dark blue sky was clear except for a few large white cumulus clouds clinging to the peaks of the Tetons. Our second day, was a shorter hike just over six miles on the Taggart Lake Trail up to Bradley Lake and back under another clear blue sky. The trails were busy with hikers, but we still managed to run across a moose grazing on the edge of the lake, and like

everyone else, we slowly and quietly crossed the bridge, stopping to watch her as she watched us. She was massive and much bigger than the moose we had encountered in the Boundary Waters. I snapped a few pictures to show the girls before the moose turned her back on us and resumed plucking marsh grasses from the shallow lake bottom. It was a short trip that year because of family obligations, but it was by far the most rewarding. I was 10 years older, but I was back to holding my own.

The first morning home from Jackson Hole, I sat on the screened in porch, taking in the sights and sounds. A yellow finch twittered through the locust branches in our front yard. The sunlight caught the whisper of a spider's shimmering silver strands lacing the dying branches of the adjacent pine tree as it swayed on a gentle breeze. The morning air was speckled with floating particles and our freshly mowed lawn outlined the wild landscape, preparing for its winter slumber. The sunlight dappled the ground as it moved through the limbs of the maple tree, revealing a bumble bee, seemingly lost as it searched for nectar. A chattering squirrel leapt from tree to tree across the open yard, and a bunny hopped out of the prairie to nibble the fresh cut grass. Mindfulness had opened me to the surrounding beauty and the ability to appreciate even the brightly painted yellow and black argiope spider living outside of our garage as it repaired its broken web.

In the beginning of my battle, there was much talk about adopting the "new normal" after cancer treatment. Generally, the reference was to the negative impacts cancer treatment would inevitably have on me, but I rejected that notion. With a full decade passed, I have grown to understand that the term "new normal" didn't necessarily have to refer to a "normal" of pain, emotional strife and fear. The "new normal" could also mean the "new normal of cancer treatment," which included a variety of modalities and practices to heal the whole patient. My "new normal" was filled with meditation, mindfulness and a deeper understanding of how to find my life's path. I have no way of knowing if I would've gotten there on my own, so for that I am grateful to have battled. In the end, Darcy was right. I was buying time but not to die. I was buying time to learn what I needed to know to transform.

"I began to have an idea of my life, not as the slow shaping of achievement to fit my preconceived purposes, but as the gradual discovery and growth of a purpose which I did not know." Joanna Field, 1900 English psychology

The End

EAT WITH THE INTENTION TO HEAL®

Fruits
Apple
Blackberry
Black Raspberry
Blueberry
Cranberry
Currant
Grapefruit
Lemons
Melon
Orange
Pineapple
Pear
Peach
Plum
Raspberry
Red Grape
Red Tart Cherry
Strawberry
Watermelon

Herbs
Basil
Chive
Cilantro
Dill
Garlic
Ginger
Fenugreek
Lavender
Licorice
Marjoram
Mint
Nutmeg
Oregano
Parsley
Rosemary
Thyme
Turmeric w/pepper
Sage

Vegetables
Artichoke
Arugula
Asparagus
Beet
Bok Choy
Brussel Sprout
Broccoli
Cabbage
Carrots
Cauliflower
Celeriac
Celery
Collard
Cucumber
Fennel
Green Bean
Kale
Leek
Lima Bean
Maitake Mushroom
Mesclun
Onion

Vegetables
Parsnip
Pea
Pepper
Pumpkin
Purple Potato
Pumpkin
Radish
Rutabaga
Scallion
Shallot
Soy Bean
Spinach
Swiss Chard
Squash
Sweet Potato
Tomato
Turnip
Watercress

Proteins
Grass-fed Chicken
Grass-fed Turkey
Grass-fed Eggs
Wild Caught Sea Food
Grass-fed Beef (limit)
Grass-fed Pork (limit)

Nuts
Almonds
Brazil Nuts
Hazelnuts
Walnuts

Other
Dark Chocolate (70+%)
Green Tea
Red Wine (1 glass/wk)
Grape Seed Oil
Olive Oil
Black Raspberry Extract
Kalonji Oil

Eat with the intention to heal.

www.kathymydlachbero.com

Acknowledgements

I have such deep gratitude for everyone who encouraged me to write this book before I could even imagine anyone would want to read it. They helped me discover that I didn't just *want* to write my story, I *needed* to write it. Even so, I never could've completed the project if not for the blind support of my parents, MaryJo and Don Mydlach. Without their non-judgmental encouragement for whatever I chose to do, I might not have believed in myself enough to beat cancer, start an organization and tell my story to anyone who would listen. I stand in awe of their deep love and willingness to drop anything and everything in their own lives to take care of me and my family. There are no words to express my love for them.

When it comes to Ron, Hannah and EmmaGrace, I have no idea how hard it was for them to have a mom and a wife battling a deadly disease, and they will likely never know the depth of my gratitude for their enduring love despite how unlovable I became. Helping us all cope were our various pets from Simon's discovery to Kie, Albert, Jack and Skip's watchful eyes over us at-all-times, offering entertaining antics, soft warm fur to stroke and unconditional love.

I am also deeply grateful to Suzannah Bong, my sister-in-law, who trusted her gut and didn't let me fall through the cracks of blind trust in the medical profession. Offering loving support and on-call child care, my in-laws Ron and Mary Bero played a crucial role in managing our family during cancer treatment. And to the rest of my family who found the time to support their ailing sibling in one way or another - Phil and Jo Mydlach, Karen Locher, Amy and Zak Stigler, Matt, Mike and Sarah Bero and Rick and Jane Bero – thank you!

Friendships came and went during my battle, but I am so grateful to those whose kindness and support carried me through the morass, particularly Camron Davis, Katelyn Varhely, Larry Mullen, Jr., Ann Acheson, Debbie O'Reilly Christiansen, Mary Krause, Lisa and Bob Conley, Jill Bedford, Sheila Young, Danelle O'Neill, Karen Allen, Ann Fredrich and Dawn Palmer. I can't forget Dave Evans "The Edge" without whom Larry wouldn't have heard about anti-angiogenesis. His willingness to share what he knew, greatly increased my chance of survival. There are many others who have passed from this world but not before they touched my soul, and my heart still aches for them.

Jack Losso, Gary Stoner and Steve Dunfield became new friends during the most difficult time in my life when they embraced me in my quest for something better. I love you guys and your humble commitment to using food as medicine. Your strength to invest in this work is not necessarily lucrative, but I know it is incredibly satisfying for you. I am entirely confident that your work will eventually make life a whole lot easier for so many suffering from chronic disease, and I am blessed to know you. As far as researchers go, I would be remiss not to mention the late Dr. David Servan-Schreiber who accidentally discovered he had cancer during a research project and eventually went on to write his pioneering book *ANTI-CANCER: A New Way Of Life,* which became my bible of sorts.

I am also grateful to the staff at Commonweal in Bolinas, California, whose program of compassionate action saved my psyche and opened my heart to abandon the detour I was on and realign myself with my life's mission. My medical team went above and beyond their defined protocol, embracing my "proactive" ways. Dr. Anne Tousignant always advocated for her patients even when her peers made it difficult. Dr. Chris Davies, Dr. Ron Fickle, Dr. Mary Fox, Dr. Kay Klaas, Dr. Rich Hansen and Physical Therapist Kathy Bussen were all key members of my team and graciously never made me feel crazy for pursuing something outside the norm. I especially want to thank Dr. Dave Rakel who helped me shed prescription medications, catapulting my recovery while validating my desire to pursue energy work and self-healing. Dr. Rakel encouraged me to step back from NuGenesis "for my own good" and to be courageous when I told my story, making sure not to sugar coat anything. I think I succeeded, Dave. The folks at Tobins Pharmacy, especially Dave, Colleen and Anya, were my shepherds through the process of supplement use, helping me avoid wasting time, energy and money. I still trust their excellent advice as I work towards a full recovery. Finally, after Ron and I closed our family gardens down, we found Paul and Laura Phelps, proprieters of Serenity Farm, an organic CSA (Community Supported Agriculture). We are so grateful for their hard work and are lucky to be able to call them friends.

My audacious belief that I could help others while still trying to help myself was shunned by many but not Ford Titus. I have never met anyone with such a strong visionary perspective for community-wide corporate responsibility. His team took my ideas and ran with them, helping me start the first-of-its-kind organization dedicated to teaching how to use food as medicine. I want to especially thank Claire O'Sheel, Matt Wade, Kathy Strombohm and Kathryn Leverenz along with the first NuGenesis Board who trusted in my passion to bring a new kind of hope to patients everywhere. To the nearly 1,000 volunteers who gave their blood, sweat and tears to lift NuGenesis and help it soar, I can never thank you enough. While I couldn't meet every one of you, I tried and am a better person knowing you and how you honored yourself and your loved ones by serving others.

254

At the beginning of the writing process, I had deep doubts about my abilities to write anything let alone a book until Camron Davis and Sheila Young took a quick read through my first 50 pages. It was their compassionately honest critiques that encouraged me to keep writing, pointing out my book wasn't just for me. When my manuscript was completed, it was Ann Garvin, a fellow author and wonderfully sardonic friend, who provided me with praise and tactful admonishment as she coached me to rework some of my writing. Also, My gratitude goes to my long-time friend Sue Schneidler who combed through the punctuation and grammar I had forgotten since journalism school. When I was ready for a publisher, I threw a desperate prayer up to the heavens that was met with what might've seemed like a random run in with an old friend, Chip Duncan, in the halls of the cancer center. Without his decisive intervention, I'd probably still be sitting at my desk wasting away as I waded through the myriad lists of agents and publishers, hoping to find a match for my book. With unequivocal confidence, Chip introduced me to "someone he knew" and within three days Bill Gladstone, owner of Waterside Productions, sent me a contract. Only hours after I received the contract, Entertainment Attorney Margaret Lund magically appeared to review it while I stood as if a deer in the headlights, trying to figure out how I could see an old friend, be introduced to a publisher, secure an entertainment attorney and have a signed contract all in three short days.

In closing, I also thank all of you who have read my book, and I hope you got something useful out of it.

ENDORSEMENTS

Kathy Bero's health journey is simply remarkable. It gives a glimpse into the dynamic healing potential of human beings and offers direction for anyone wanting to navigate the key ingredients of one's powerful self-healing mechanisms. This book helps us learn from an outlier that found a healing path when our science did not think it was possible. It gives hope of a better life, no matter the outcome.

David Rakel MD, FAAFP, Founder and Director, University of Wisconsin Integrative Medicine, Professor and Chair, Department of Family & Community Medicine, University of New Mexico School of Medicine, Albuquerque, NM

From her perspective as a mother, a daughter, and a wife fighting an epic battle for her life, Kathy Bero weaves a beautifully crafted story. Based on a deep dive into her journals, this is a moving and inspiring heroine's journey that is a learning opportunity for everyone, even if you don't have cancer.

Linda Sechrist, Senior Staff Writer for Natural Awakenings

It was my great pleasure and privilege to meet Kathy Bero a few years ago while serving as a faculty member of the Medical College of Wisconsin. Kathy told me about her personal health challenges and how she was addressing them by not only standard clinical treatment, but also, by eating healthy foods that we all know contain compounds that are important for disease prevention and treatment. Indeed, it was remarkable how she withstood serious disease by consuming healthy foods, which led to her to live by the motto: "Food is Your Medicine." With me, she is preaching to the choir, as I have spent much of my career examining the disease preventive effects of different foods. Her role in establishing NuGenesis Farm was one major step she has taken to implement her beliefs. Writing this book is another. Let's all join Kathy in her efforts to encourage the eating of quality foods for our health and happiness!

Sincerely, Gary Stoner, PhD, Director of the Molecular Carcinogenesis and Chemoprevention Program Professor of Medicine, Hematology and Oncology, Medical College of Wisconsin, Professor Emeritus, Department of Internal Medicine, Ohio State University

From the moment I met Kathy, I was inspired. Her positivity, energy and passion are simply contagious. Kathy's deep belief in being your own advocate empowered her fight and moves her each day through the journey of her beautiful life. Her story is sure to make you realize the power of believing in yourself!

Bridget Clementi (personal endorsement)
Retired NuGenesis Board Member Vice-President, Community Health at Children's Hospital of Wisconsin

Made in the USA
Middletown, DE
31 January 2019